I'll
Start
Again
Tomorrow

I'll Start Again Tomorrow

And Other Lies I've Told Myself

SONIA JHAS

●● PAGE TWO

Cataloguing in publication information is
available from Library and Archives Canada.

ISBN 978-1-77458-312-8 (paperback)
ISBN 978-1-77458-313-5 (ebook)
ISBN 978-1-77458-314-2 (audiobook)

Page Two
pagetwo.com

Copyedited by Melissa Kawaguchi and Kendra Ward
Cover and interior design by Jennifer Lum
Cover photo by Gooseberry Studios

soniajhas.com

Contents

A Note from Me to You

I WANT TO BE CLEAR before we dive in together: the contents of this book do not constitute professional therapy or medical advice.

I love this book. I'm proud of this book. I'm *so* glad you've found this book. But I also know that this book is *not* the same as seeking professional help for your mental and physical health. So as happy as I am that you've decided to pick up this book, please don't go into it thinking that it holds all the answers for a "cure." It doesn't. Instead, think of this book as an honest, friendly (hopefully amusing) companion on your path toward healing.

I'm about to share many of my raw, personal experiences with you. My hope is that you'll learn from my missteps so that when you make your own mistakes (and yes, you *will* make mistakes), you're able to course-correct with more empathy and compassion. As you make your way through this book, notice what resonates with you and internalize the lessons that feel important. If anything brings up self-destructive thoughts, skip past it. No really, I give you full permission to do that. This isn't meant to be painful.

I know that the path to healing isn't as simple as a quick read, some slick calorie math, and a series of organized work-outs. It's complicated and non-linear. As you'll see in the pages that follow, my journey has been a long and winding road with too many detours and U-turns to count. And my journey *still* continues because there is no final destination. There is no finish line. There is no certificate that says, "I'm healed forever."

It's an ongoing process to rise above the noise, to rely on the tools and skills you develop, to stay committed to the path of healing. But healing *is* possible if you get the support you need. For me, therapy has been and continues to be a core component of my journey.

With love,
Sonia

Introduction

CONGRATULATIONS ON TAKING THE FIRST step to upgrading your mindset, your lifestyle, and your relationship with your body. I know the journey to this point hasn't been easy for you. I get it.

No, trust me.

I get it.

I know you probably had to leverage a lot of self-talk and will-power to crack this book open. Sure, I bet you were excited when you bought it, but I also know firsthand that it would have been much easier for you to listen to the voice in your head telling you to curl up on the sofa with Netflix.

I applaud you for listening to the other, more aggressive, voice in your head semi-yelling at you, "Just shut the hell up and read the damn book because it's time to overcome your bullshit once and for all!" It would have been way easier to shut that voice up with some mindless social media scrolling, or a snack, or better yet mindless social media scrolling *with* many snacks because, let's face it, when is that not a winning combo?

And yet here you are.
You made it.
Well done.

Now, close your eyes for a second. I want you to think back to your childhood. Really live there for a moment. I want you to see the colors vividly, hear the laughter in your ears, and feel the sense of freedom wash over you. Okay, maybe that's a bit dramatic, but at the very least I want you to remember what it felt like to be a child. It was a simpler time, wasn't it? A time when you felt uninhibited. A time when you felt unburdened. A time when you felt free.

I remember riding my bike outside for hours on end (for the sheer pleasure of it, *not* because cardio can help you shed fat). I remember eating popsicles until my teeth changed color (without thinking about how many calories I'd already eaten that day). I remember performing cute little dance numbers to the entire *Dance Mix '93* soundtrack (without worrying whether people could see my body jiggle while I did the "running man").

Most of us start our lives off as happy, confident kids. And then somewhere along the way, for one set of reasons or another, life starts to chip away at our freedom. We forget what it's like to feel uninhibited, unburdened, and free, both mentally and physically, because we're dealing with *real things* like finances, careers, relationships, and *things that feel like real things*, like social media. Most importantly, we become preoccupied with the idea of squeezing ourselves into molds (like skinny jeans) that don't quite fit. We filter ourselves. We lose authenticity on the quest to gain likes and followers, and somewhere along the way we lose touch with who we really are.

Chasing beauty.
Chasing success.
Chasing happiness.
Chasing ... period.
And holy shit, is it ever exhausting.

Now, because you're reading this book, I'm going to go ahead and assume that at some point or another you've committed to becoming better, stronger, more connected with yourself, more at peace. Even if you haven't tried to jump on the official fitness bandwagon, I'm willing to bet that there have been moments in your life (like every single January 1st since elementary school) when you've told yourself that you're "officially" going to start

- eating healthier,
- being more physically active,
- meditating,
- being more positive, or
- writing in a gratitude journal.

I know I'm not the only one who's spent her life trying to "suck less" year after year. We've all made attempts at some version of an "improvement journey." In fact, if you're anything like me, you've probably come at the "how do I fix myself" problem time and time again from various angles only to find yourself back at the starting point. Maybe your strategies worked for a short period of time—a week, a month, six months, or even a year. But for most of you, long-term sustainable change has probably felt next to impossible.

I've been there.

I get it.

Like many women out there, I spent most of my youth on the hamster wheel of weight loss. For Indian people, the expectation around female beauty involves some combination of "enough meat on your bones" (without being too meaty) and "voluptuous curves" (without being too voluptuous). Muscle definition is considered anything but feminine, and being too skinny is a sign that your parents or husband aren't feeding you properly. I don't buy into this narrative, obviously, but it did create many layers of confusion for me while growing up. And body-image issues? Oh God, I had plenty. And to think, this was all before Instagram came into the mix. A simpler time when I was only being compared to all 850 of our family friends.

I used to be your classic "on the wagon, off the wagon" kind of girl. On the first Monday of every month, I would declare to myself and others (because what's life without the added pressure of judgment) that I

- was in it to win it,
- wouldn't make the same mistakes as before,
- would do better . . . be better . . . live better!

And yet, no matter how hard I'd try, I'd always slip. Just a little at first. Then a full-fledged rebound. I don't think my story is unique. I feel like most women have lived some version of it.

The question is, why?

Why do we do this to ourselves?

What are we really striving for?

Is the crux of the issue the problem statement itself: "How do I fix myself?" (Hint: yes, it is.)

And do the journey and the outcome shift when we change the language to: "Who is it that I'm trying to be and what's stopping me from getting there?" (Hint: yes, they do.)

My earliest memory of playing the body comparison game dates back to 1994—when I was nine years old and in the fourth grade. Spandex shorts and bodysuits were all the rage, and even though I was young, I wanted to fit in and wear the cool-kid outfits. So, there I was one day, sitting at my desk, wearing my newest bodysuit. I don't remember what my teacher was talking about, but I *do* remember the exact moment I looked down at my lap and thought, "Oh, wow, look at how big your stomach looks! It's not flat. It's totally round and sticking out. Eww." You see, even at that age, I was coveting the perfection my culture expected and the perfection (I thought) the world expected. Had anyone ever called me fat before? No. Had anyone ever told me that my stomach was supposed to look flat? No. And yet there I was, at the age of nine, suddenly unimpressed with myself. I remember feeling embarrassed and disappointed. I remember thinking, "What do I do to fix this?" At that moment I tried something I had never done before: I sucked in my stomach and kept it contracted without holding my breath. My stomach was flat. My "problem" was gone. I looked instantly thinner, and I loved it. And that's when it all started . . . when I realized that I looked better with my stomach sucked in (at least in my mind), and if I remained conscious of it, I could make sure I always looked like that. I kept it a secret. My flat stomach made me feel special, like I had something everyone else wanted.

That day in fourth grade began the next eighteen years of my life, in which not a single day went by that I let my stomach loose. Years of performing, slowly detaching myself from the dull, achy fatigue that comes from contracting your core (and your soul) day in and day out. But it felt worth it. People noticed and commented on my physique, cementing a belief, a mindset, a way of being in the world that would later take me years to unlayer and unlearn. When I think back to this time, I can see so clearly where all of my "chasing" began.

So preoccupied with how others saw me.

So concerned with how I measured up.

So wrapped up in the narrative that "thin equals happy" before I had even gone from girl to woman.

Do you remember moments like this?

Can you pinpoint *when* the comparison seeds were planted?

Can you *feel* how the moments shaped you into who you have become today?

Are you *ready* to let it all go for something more freeing?

Even as adults, we continue to perpetuate the cycle. Taking picture after picture hoping that in the *next* shot our bodies will look perfectly snatched. Contorting ourselves into awkward poses just to make sure we look as good as the random influencers. Going on diet after diet because apparently happiness is just ten pounds away and if we can get there, like all the other "beautiful people" online, then maybe, just maybe, we'll finally feel good in our own skin.

We know better, and yet we can't seem to execute life any other way until we're so exhausted from all the misaligned action and failed attempts that we have no choice but to either break free or numb the pain with distractions like food, alcohol, or (my personal favorite) Netflix and a bag of spicy popcorn.

The fact is this: We're now living in a #hashtag world. A world that is defining happiness for us, shifting our reference points on success, and causing us to question every bit of who we really are. A world that is flattening us to one moment, one identity, one frame, and one pose. A world that is pushing us to lose the nuance of what it means to be human and preventing us from finding the beauty in the struggle of *real* life. A world so powerful that it can reduce a person's whole existence to a single post that is either validated or invalidated based solely on engagement. The filters, the highlight reels, the five-minute recipes, the lettuce "chips" that are nothing more than sad-looking pieces of air-fried lettuce—they're blurring our vision and playing with our emotions, convincing us that if we just try a *little harder,* then we, too, can achieve the ideal body. The #hashtag world has us convinced that we're "doing the work" every time we "like and save" workouts, recipes, and motivational quotes. It has us convinced that we're "doing the work" every time we decide to go keto, or do a juice cleanse, or buy another quick-fix cream. It has us convinced that we're "doing the work" every time we pretend to love the latest healthy TikTok trend, like keto sandwiches that are really just salads folded up.

But you know as well as I do that this isn't the work you need to be doing. You know as well as I do that hovering at the surface of life without doing the hard, internal work is what's keeping you stuck on the hamster wheel of weight loss . . . on the hamster wheel of life. It's *why* you can't achieve sustainable change when it comes to your mindset, your lifestyle, and your relationship with your body.

Here's the deal: I know it's tempting and frankly easy AF to stay at the surface level of life, where memes and reels pacify your angst. But if you want change—like, you *really* want it—then it's time to go deeper. It's time to stop chasing a version of perfection that you accidentally agreed upon when you didn't know any better, only to be killing the magic of who you really are along the way.

Because it doesn't have to be this way, and you don't *deserve* to feel this way.

I learned that I could choose differently, and so can you.

Throughout this book, my goal is to teach you the fundamental mindset shifts that are required to get you back in the driver's seat of your life so that you can finally break free from the "on again, off again" cycle and achieve your health and wellness goals. And please note: I say "the driver's seat of your life" because I really *am* talking about your life. The whole thing. Not *just* your health and wellness. You're not "totally fine in all other areas of your life" but "can't seem to get your shit together when it comes to fitness and nutrition." That's not how it works. Truth be told, what's holding you back from making peace with your body is also what's holding you back in every other area of your life—your relationships, career, boundaries, choices, and desires.

Throughout this book, you'll see that I've layered in many of my own personal stories to give you a glimpse of what my *real* journey has been about. I don't want you to believe that I've just been #blessed throughout my life, that becoming who I am today has been a gentle, gradual progression, or that I've seamlessly transformed my body, my mind, and my life without struggle.

That couldn't be further from the truth.

You'll see that I'm not someone who's always had her shit together.

I've deprived myself.

I've over-exercised.

I've spent more hours than I'd like to admit doom scrolling through the #hashtag world, comparing myself to the "perfect" girls online, even though I know they aren't real.

You are not alone.

So, take a deep breath, knowing that change is possible and that it's not as complicated as it seems if you go about it the right way. When I reclaimed my body, I reclaimed my power, and that's when my whole life changed. By digging into my values, exploring my limiting beliefs, and confronting my self-sabotaging behaviors, I made it to the other side, and that's where I found freedom.

The freedom to let go of all the angst and negative narrative.

The freedom to break free from the molds I had forced myself into.

The freedom to discover who I really am.

This is my hope for you, too.

Look, I get that you may have bought this book with the (secret) hope that you were going to get the "cheat sheet" rundown on how to lose weight fast, only to now be confronted with a whole lot of mindset talk. You're either irritated or you're intrigued. I'm hoping it's the latter, because *I know* that *you know* that simply "knowing the facts about fitness and nutrition" has very little to do with your ultimate success.

You've been down that road before. Likely many times. You know you actually have to do things differently this time in order to reach a new destination. More importantly, you have to *think* differently. The truth is this: You've signed up for the hard work. This shit ain't easy. And I don't mean "not easy" in the same way running a half-marathon isn't easy. I mean "not easy" because you're now going to be embarking on a path to confront the questions that make you feel the most uncomfortable.

What do I really want?

Whose voices are stuck in my head?

Why do I feel like I'm either procrastinating or "so in it" that I can't find balance?

My hope is to walk you through these questions, and more, with intentionality and guidance because, frankly, I wish I'd had that kind of support. In my case, it felt more like I was running through chaos, arms flailing, hoping to make it to the other side. I now know that there's a better, gentler, way less dramatic path to uncovering your truest self, and that's what I'm bringing to you in the pages that follow. Commit to the journey, live through the questions I ask you, and I promise you'll come out the other side with the change, progress, and evolution you deserve.

1

Happiness Is Always
Ten Pounds Away

WHAT DO YOU *REALLY* WANT? You're likely chasing a lot of things right now—like money, beauty, prestige, and love. But *why* do you want those things? Are your goals *really* yours or are they simply a reflection of what the #hashtag world has conditioned you to believe you want?

"Once I lose the weight, then . . . I'll feel like the 'real' me."

"When my muffin top is gone, then . . . I'll stop needing to edit my pictures."

"If I just drop down a couple more dress sizes, then . . . I'll be able to sign up for that dating app."

Sound familiar? I thought so.

We're all supposed to know better by now. Obviously, it's what's on the inside that counts. Obviously, you are valuable no matter your size. Obviously, losing weight isn't going to solve all your problems. And yet, each time I give a talk, I ask my audience if they regularly have thoughts like these and, without fail, every woman in the group will raise her hand. I'm not exaggerating; literally every single woman, every single time.

I wasn't born particularly skinny, but I did learn very early on that if I made myself suffer enough, I, too, could fit into a size double zero. Sometimes I dieted. Sometimes I exercised. For the most part, I dieted and exercised. This doesn't sound all that bad, I know, but let me clarify: I'm not talking about your normal "I'm going to cut back on takeout and switch from white rice to brown rice" kind of diet. No, my diet and exercise regimen involved extreme deprivation and intense dedication.

What started out as a simple desire to drop a few pounds quickly evolved into a quiet obsession. I researched a lot:

- "Best ways to shed fat?"
- "Are carbs bad for you?"
- "Should women lift heavy weights?"

Growing up, investigating the secrets of weight loss became a (secret) hobby of mine. Yet each time I came at the problem from a different angle, I led myself straight to the same point: exceptionally hungry and on my way back to a bigger size. This cycle continued for years. Desperate to be thin, I would over-exercise and deprive myself of food only to burn myself out and rebound to my original size. Yes, everyone knows that moderation is key, but my personality is pretty type A, so moderation has never been my forte. Instead, I'd simply take time off, settle back into my comfy clothes for a while, and then start again with the vow that I'd "really stick to it this time!"

Every time I give a talk, no matter who the audience is, I get aggressive nods when I share my past. I can see that women across the room are relating with what I'm sharing because I'm speaking the truth they've been wanting to say out loud for so long: *The quest to be thin isn't just stomach-sucking, it's soul sucking*... and We're. So. Damn. Sick. Of. It.

Growing up, my entire existence was consumed by this sort of narrative:

- "When I'm a size zero, then I'll feel beautiful... "
- "Once my arms are toned, then I'll feel confident in a tank top... "
- "If I just get a little more definition in my stomach, then I'll feel like I can slow down..."

At the time, I didn't realize what I was doing to myself. I believed I was just the kind of gal who always had her eye on the prize because I was an unstoppable force dedicated to self-improvement. Sometimes it was about the number on the scale; sometimes it was about fitting into certain clothes, and sometimes it was about achieving a certain "look." Whatever the goal, I truly believed that if I wanted it badly enough and that if I could just get there somehow... then—*bam!*—I'd also arrive at happiness.

You know what's the worst, though? When you think you know what you want, but then, after it's all said and done, it turns out that you were wrong. You know when you've got your mind set on this one thing that you believe is going to make you happy and then after slogging away to get it, it just... doesn't?

Yes, *that* is the absolute worst.

And it's confusing, too, because it's hard to tell what the issue is.

Is it that you don't know yourself all that well?

Is it that you're miscalculating your desires?

Is it that you're just kind of flakey?

When it comes to changing your body, you know as well as I do that nothing happens overnight once you're past the age of... well, eighteen. Actually morphing your body—whether that means losing weight, gaining muscle, or a combination of both—requires commitment. It's the type of thing you must strap yourself in for because it's always a turbulent ride filled with speed bumps and detours.

Sometimes, no matter what you do, you just can't seem to accomplish your body goals. It feels too challenging, something else takes priority, or the Universe has other plans in store for you.

Life: it happens.

Then sometimes, you do start to progress. You start to lose the weight. You see hints of definition. You begin to fit into jeans that you'd sworn off for years. And then what happens? You fall off the wagon.

And finally, there are those times when you really do lose the weight. You see shadows and lines where before there were none. You build the booty. You conquer the abs. And then what happens? Nothing. There's no satisfaction. No self-celebration. Oh, you thought you were finally going to feel proud of yourself? Cute... but, no. Why? Because somewhere along the way, when you realized that you would achieve your goal, you unknowingly set your sights on something else.

And just like that... *happiness remains ten pounds away.*

SHAPE-SHIFTING GOALS

Here is how you got to where you are: You launched yourself hard and fast into a new diet or exercise regimen because you wanted to achieve a specific goal, like losing ten pounds or achieving ab definition, only to find that your goal began to shift the moment you started to get into a groove and make real progress. Without realizing it, you decided to tweak your goal, take it up a notch, or even take a subtle right turn to an adjacent goal. Then, instead of recognizing and feeling the progress you made toward your original goal, you were left sprinting toward a new goal, feeling nothing but uncertainty and angst along the way.

Looking back, I can see that the pattern of shape-shifting goals started early in my life, well before I began chasing the "perfect" body. In elementary school, I remember thinking that I'd be *so happy* once I got all As on my report card. In high school, I remember thinking that I'd feel *so good* once I got into a top tier university. In university, it was all about making it onto the dean's list and getting the best job because then I'd feel *so proud* of myself. Each time I knocked off an achievement, my criteria changed.

How could I be so clear about my desires and be willing to work super-hard for them, only to find myself wanting something else when I reached the finish line?

The cycle happened so many times that at a certain point I just couldn't deny it anymore. When I started to peel back the layers, I could see that I liked the feeling of wanting something. That feeling kept me motivated and determined to keep going. The race, the grueling effort, the uncertainty and anxiety about whether I would be good enough to "get there"—as counter-intuitive as it sounds, all of it made me feel right at home. And so, any time it seemed like I was getting close to achieving a goal, I would unknowingly set my sights on something bigger and better to keep me in that high-performance, subtle-anxiety-ridden state.

We all want so badly to "get there," but where is "there" when the target keeps moving? Where is "there" when our desires keep changing based on what we see in the #hashtag world? We can't even stay in our own lanes anymore. Now, we want to be the best at it all. We see someone juggling motherhood impeccably, and we think, "Oh shit, I gotta try harder!" We see someone becoming an astronaut, and we think, "Oh shit, I could have done that, too, if I had known earlier!" An entrepreneur sells their company for big money, and we think, "Oh shit, I'm never going to be able to keep up!" when we're not even in the same industry.

I did this for years. Relationships . . . my career . . . especially my body.

Somewhere along the way:

- "I want to lose weight" would turn into "It's not enough. Now I want to have a flat stomach."

- "I want to have a flat stomach" would turn into "It's not enough. Now I want to have visible abs."

- "I want to have visible abs" would turn into "It's not enough. Now I want to have a six-pack."

Sometimes the goals themselves weren't even that import-ant to me. They were just things to channel my attention toward, things to focus and ground me. Being goal-oriented had become such a habitual state for me that I felt like I had no identity without the "am I good enough to achieve?" narrative.

But how do you get to know yourself when you're compar-ing who you are, what you look like, and what you've achieved with everyone in the entire world? How do you get to know the *real you* when you're so busy presenting the #hashag ver-sion of yourself to the world, based on what you assume people want to see?

My goals often morphed based on other people. I'd find myself mesmerized by someone I respected who had achieved something really great, and just like that, I'd unknowingly shift my goals to look a little more like their list of achieve-ments. Someone had a particularly tiny waist? Suddenly, I wanted that, too. Someone ran a half-marathon? Now I needed to add that to the list. Someone landed a higher-paying job? Oh, you bet that went on my radar as well.

Who was I without goals hanging over my head? Why was I so afraid of not having something to work toward? Would it always be a game of "more?" Would I ever be content? And if what I was working toward was always evolving into some-thing else, then what was my motivation really based on? What did I really value?

THE ANTICLIMACTIC WIN

Most of my wins in life felt anticlimactic. I'd make it to the end of the journey, hold my head up high, and feel a brief moment of relief—followed by some version of "Sure, I'm happy, I guess, but really, it's no big deal . . . Once I achieve 'blah blah blah,' then I'll really feel like I've made it." It happened time and time again, whether about my body or my life achievements. Every time I lost the weight, all I wanted was to lose more. I lost ten pounds? Suddenly, that felt like no big deal because it's common for people to lose ten pounds. Now, to feel really proud of myself, I needed a set of abs to go with my new look. I'd never admit this out loud, of course, but in my mind, I knew that whatever I had achieved just wasn't enough. The cycle was always the same: all the work, all the buildup, with nothing but mild letdown at the end.

All I really felt was longing for something more.

Each time it happened, I'd convince myself that what I really needed were more goals, better goals, *more aggressive* goals. However, the problems lay not with my goals but with my value system.

NO BULLSHIT PLATITUDES

If you're chasing a dream that feels far off in the distance, like finally losing twenty pounds, and you think that getting to that promised land will make you feel the way you want to feel, then let me cut to the chase and share one of the hardest lessons I've learned in my life: There is no promised land. There is only *right here, right now.*

I know, I know. This sounds like all those other vague Insta-quotes you're used to reading. You know the ones I mean, like:

- "Wherever you go, there you are."
- "You have to look through the rain to see the rainbow."
- "Live. Laugh. Love."

Yes, the platitudes that float around the #hashtag world. The quotes that simultaneously calm us down and create more angst because while they kind of mean something, they mostly mean nothing, and we don't know what to do with them. We *want* to feel better because they're technically reassuring words, but all we really feel is more damaged and alone.

But hear me out. No bullshit platitudes here. I promise this will be worth your while.

Creating specific goals for yourself can be a strategic step to achieving the outcomes you're looking for in life, especially when it comes to your body. I'm a big believer in setting smart, realistic, actionable goals. However, if you're not careful, creating goals can also serve as comfortable busy-work that keeps you from doing the uncomfortable *real work.* You know, the messy soul stuff like looking inward, understanding what really matters to you, clarifying your motivation, and most importantly, finding joy along the way. Here's the deal: the reason losing weight or getting fit or achieving the body of your dreams feels both overwhelming during the journey and underwhelming when you achieve success is because you don't know what really matters to you.

When asked, most people will say that their primary focus when embarking on a new fitness or nutrition regimen is to feel a renewed sense of health and vitality. And of course, that answer will always get a roaring 10/10 score. But is it true? Are most people really after health and vitality? Is that what your journey has really been about so far? Or . . .

- Is it about gaining respect from others and hearing it in the form of admiration and praise?
- Is it about finally feeling more beautiful?
- Is it about proving to yourself that you're disciplined and focused?

Whether you're the kind of person who struggles to stay on track with fitness and nutrition for more than a couple of months or you're the type who sticks to the plan until you achieve your goals only to fall off the wagon shortly afterward, the first step in your journey is the same: you must clarify what's really driving you.

QUIT THE CHASE

When you fail to uncover what really matters to you at your core (and to be clear, that's not what you think is "supposed" to matter to you), you're simply flying blind on this journey of life, hoping that something like losing weight will do the trick, and usually it doesn't. In fact, when you're out of touch with what you really want in life, you're often working at cross-purposes with what you really need.

I spent years of my life trekking to the tops of mountains. Sometimes I'd be defeated along the way because I simply couldn't cut it. Let's be real here: nobody's becoming a doctor or engineer if they suck at chemistry and physics. In other cases, I'd make it to the summit only to realize that I was at the wrong peak. If you're like me, guilty of achieving goals that ultimately don't lead to happiness, it's safe to say your goals are misaligned with your core self and it's time for a major point of integration.

Let me give you a few examples of how I spent years missing the truth of who I really am and what I really cared about:

- **Body.** I was striving to be skinny when what I really needed was to feel strong, fit, and full of vitality.

- **Self-worth.** I was striving to be perfect when what I really needed was to feel confident and good in my own skin, as is.

- **Career.** I was striving for a high-paying corporate job when what I really needed was to experience inspiration and fulfillment in a calling that was uniquely my own.

Once upon a time, I thought I was following an unconventional path by getting a commerce degree. I know that sounds totally ridiculous; I'm talking about a prestigious degree at a top tier university, not running off to tame lions (although that does sound kind of cool). But when you're raised by Indian parents whose only hope is that you'll grow up to become an engineer or a doctor, getting a business degree is considered pretty risqué. Particularly when you have an older brother who managed to become both an engineer *and* a doctor.

But yes, I chose the unbeaten path of studying commerce at university, and despite a brief stint on academic probation because of my inability to effectively understand

Accounting 101, I successfully clawed my way through four years of undergrad, graduated on the dean's list, and accepted an incredible offer to start my career in an executive position at IBM.

On paper, things looked pretty sweet for me. I had twisted myself into a perfect pretzel, I was succeeding to the level of everyone else's standards, and I was living some version of "the dream."

Yet the perfectionist in me constantly wanted more.

After every achievement, I'd feel glorified for a split second, but then I'd feel untethered without another challenge to face. Something about my job at IBM left me feeling unfulfilled and kind of like a fraud, so I knew the job wasn't going to cut it in the long run, despite the great money. Was it that I didn't like technology? Was it that I felt like I had no real skills to bring to the table? Was it that I felt like I didn't belong in the environment? I suspect it was some combination of all of the above. So, at the age of twenty-six, I decided to pursue my MBA in the hopes that it would answer the whole "what am I meant to do with my life?" dilemma.

While doing my MBA, I also purchased a home and planned and executed my wedding to a man who had just started his neurosurgical residency training. Moderation? As I said earlier, that shit has never been my forte.

I kept adding challenge after challenge to my already high-stress life because I was hungry for something more. I continued to find ways to chase more, and when there was nothing left, I desperately chased the idea of being "skinny." Very quickly, the gym became my happy place. I started eating well (or so I thought at the time), I trained hard (too hard), and I loved the progress that I was making (because my clothes started to get looser). I felt stronger than ever, I felt more intense than ever, and I was thriving off those endorphins.

Until it happened—my first grown-up rebound. I should have known my streak wouldn't last, because I had all the classic symptoms of burnout. Perma-fatigue had set in, and I ate everything in sight. No, really. I ate *all* the things. I was in ooey-gooey, cheesy, bready heaven until my skinny jeans got too tight for me to wear without muffin-topping over them.

I had been through the rebound cycle enough times to know how to get the weight off quickly, but this time around felt different. I felt like I couldn't buy my own bullshit anymore. The constant drive to chase accolades and thinness had exhausted me, and I felt utterly sick of myself. I wanted something more meaningful.

And so I decided, for the first time in my life, to look inward. I knew that if I wanted to be more, do more, live more, and love myself more that I would have to stop Band-Aid-solutioning my life and start digging through the dirt of who I was. What did that really mean? I wasn't sure. I just knew that I needed to heal the most obvious, undeniable pain point first: my body.

I started by listening to a faint whisper that slowly became louder and louder.

"I want to be healthy."

"I want to be happy."

"I want to feel good."

"I want to feel like *me*."

While I didn't realize it at the time, tuning in to the quiet whispers of my soul set me off on a journey to explore my values. I started to dig through the mess of what was driving me and my beliefs and realized that identifying my core values could help me break my constant self-hate, quick-fix cycle and finally help me get into the driver's seat of my own happiness.

When I began to peel the layers back, I discovered:

- **I valued vitality.** I wanted to nourish myself and build strength, not starve myself and run myself ragged. I wanted to learn about health and nutrition and do things the right way.

- **I valued self-love.** Sure, I wanted to be able to praise myself for toning up my arms, but I also wanted to be kind to myself in the mirror no matter what I looked like, particularly when I was struggling to keep things on track.

- **I valued alignment.** I desperately wanted to work with my body instead of constantly fighting against it.

The more I focused on these three elements, the more connected I felt to the *real* Sonia. I could feel myself shifting. It was as if by focusing on the inner work and letting it blossom outward, instead of focusing on the fake outer work, hoping that it would bleed inward, I was able to get to the core of who I am. Identifying and tuning in to my values was the first step in ending my decade-long love-hate relationship with my body, and the changes didn't end there. I quickly (but painfully) realized that my corporate career no longer aligned with what I truly wanted, and my newfound understanding gave me the courage to say goodbye to a life that wasn't serving me. Of course, there was a ton of anxiety and fear along the way, but I made the leap, and I haven't looked back.

REFLECT AND REMEMBER

Reflect

Can you take a step back from wanting to "quickly get fit" to tune in to what sparks excitement in you and (more importantly) what drains you? What resistance, if any, comes up for you when you think about doing this kind of inner work?

Remember

1. Chasing goal after goal to the point of burnout is not a sign of success. It's a clear signal that something in your life needs to be reevaluated.

2. Even though it may feel shitty to do so, it's important to take some time to reflect on your past experiences to evaluate where your motivation (or lack thereof) has been coming from.

3. Your core values are the secret to feeling your best, and if you learn to identify them, you'll be one step closer to breaking your on-again, off-again cycle.

2
Pivot Your Perspective

ONE OF MY FAVORITE WAYS to explore my values is by putting my goals aside for a moment and asking myself this extremely simple yet potent question: How do I *want* to feel?

Our feelings hold all the answers we're so badly searching for, but most of us quiet them, numb them, or suppress them because it's easier to be in "doing mode" than "feeling mode," especially when you're a go-getter who needs results.

DOING MODE	FEELING MODE
I must go to the gym six days a week and work out for ninety minutes each session.	I'm tired; my body needs rest and recovery. This feels really hard.
I must eat fewer than one thousand calories a day, cut out all carbs, and avoid all fat.	I feel fatigued, hungry, and foggy. I need to nourish myself.
I'm going to sign up for a half-marathon this summer.	I seriously kind of hate running.

Despite what it may look like, the point of "feeling mode" isn't for us to succumb to our lazier selves but rather to show us the power and value of our feelings so that we can make healthy lifestyle choices that don't feel so incredibly soul-sucking in the long run.

Whenever I begin working with a new client, I ask them what they believe their greatest struggle is when it comes to health and wellness. Most often, "motivation" is the answer. However, when I start to peel back the layers, all too often I find that they're trying to be "motivated" about things that they actually kind of hate, like eating super-low-calorie meals that taste like cardboard or drinking celery juice. Is it that they're unmotivated, or is it that the things they're asking themselves to do *feel* pretty shitty?

For a long time, doing came far more naturally to me than feeling. I played the part of the perfect little Indian girl for too many years, keeping my opinions to myself. I learned at an early age that this was the expected code of conduct, and I played the role pretty damned well, all the way into adulthood. My parents were traditional. Like any stereotypical Indian family, we had to follow the standard principles (what I call the "ticky marks"):

TICKY MARKS	TRANSLATION
Do well in school.	90-plus percent only . . . and even still, they'll ask, "What happened to the other 10 percent?"
Don't talk to boys.	Don't even look at them until it's time to get married.
Respect your elders.	Follow them blindly without ever questioning, "Why?"
Don't swear.	Even the word "stupid" is off-limits.
Don't wear slutty clothes.	Nothing tight, nothing short, nothing on-trend.

For those of you who don't know, there's also a follow-up list that includes some very binary indicators of success:

- Get married to a successful Indian boy or a fair-skinned Indian girl.
- Get a postgraduate degree to legitimize yourself if it takes too long to get married.
- Make a six-figure salary to legitimize yourself if you're not already a doctor, lawyer, or engineer.
- Buy a large home.
- Have many babies.

But my parents' list of ticky marks wasn't quite so short. They had other unstated expectations about everything. Growing up in my parents' household:

- We did not watch too much TV or have the TV on in the background while doing other things.
- We did not sleep in, even on the weekends (seriously, my dad would start vacuuming at 7:30 a.m. to ensure we were up and at 'em).
- We did not keep junk food in the house, and when we did occasionally eat junk food, it was to be done in extreme moderation.

As if these somewhat militant rules weren't hard enough for a girl who just wanted to be an average kid, there was also a set of unspoken rules about feelings:

- Don't talk too loudly or too much.
- Don't express negative feelings.
- Don't talk about things that feel uncomfortable, hard, or scary.

In a nutshell, I learned that I wasn't supposed to talk about feelings at all.

If all those restrictions and expectations sound limiting to you, rest assured my therapist agrees. And I don't think I'm unique. There are probably a lot of you who feel like you had to deal with restrictive ticky marks as children. Sadly, these ticky marks shape so much of how we perceive and conduct ourselves when we grow up. It's no wonder so many of us struggle to connect with our true desires and feelings.

Most people rarely pause to consider what it truly means to achieve success in their own lives—from their body to their relationships, from family to money to career. But your values, and yours alone, hold the answers to questions like: "Why can't I really feel happy with my body?" "When will I get to the point where I genuinely feel proud of myself?" "When will I feel truly comfortable in my own skin, regardless of how many likes I get online?"

If you feel like your own dreams and desires are buried way down, like mine were, then *now* is the time to tap into your core self and revive them. It's time to stop climbing the wrong ladders to someone else's version of beauty, health, and success, and to start defining your own messy but beautiful path.

I know you probably know this, but let's start with a basic refresher so that I'm confident we're all on the same page before we move forward.

GETTING TO THE CORE

Values are your fundamental beliefs, an internal representation of what is most important to you at your deepest, core level. They're your principles or standards of behavior, your judgment of what is important in life. Values have a major influence on your attitude and behavior and serve as broad guidelines in all situations. They determine what you do with your time and how you evaluate the time you spend. Unlike your goals, which exist in the future, your values exist in the present moment. In an ideal scenario, they are freely chosen *by you*, not imposed *on you* by external sources.

It's all about what matters most to you.

Read that again and sit with it for a moment because it's absolutely crucial.

Like I did, you probably have some work to do when it comes to identifying your own core values. Sure, you may not have grown up with Indian parents, but I suspect that the #hashtag world has made your vision just as blurry as mine used to be. I know this may sound like annoying homework, but it's also an exciting place to be. It takes many people years and years to even get here, to be able to recognize that they're not living in alignment. And let me just say that once you get through the work, you'll truly gain more clarity in your life.

Values drive our goals, our decisions, and our actions. If we don't know what's important to us, we spend a lot of time wondering what in the hell we should be doing.

Do you find yourself constantly asking yourself questions like:

"Why can't I lose the weight and keep it off for good?"

"Why do I keep falling off the wagon?"

"Why can't I stay motivated?"

Wasted energy.

So much angst.

Very little gain.

When we live according to our values, we experience a sense of groundedness, calm, and peace of mind. Day-to-day choices become easier, as does life overall, and while it doesn't always stay easy—because, hello, it's life—things will feel more in harmony with who you are and what your goals are, even in the most challenging of times.

Our values drive us to spend our time in ways that support what is most important to us, and by becoming consciously aware of our values, we can use them to make more informed decisions about our health and wellness goals.

So, trust me, it's worth doing the work.

But let me remind you that this is just the beginning. Quickly coming up with a new list of values so that you can "get skinny" can't be the objective. This is about the journey, so let's make it fun, okay? Let's try to figure out how you can enjoy the process of finding out who you really are and what you really want out of life and your relationship with your body.

By identifying these deeper drivers in your life, you'll be able to figure out how they might subconsciously be shaping your behaviors and begin to understand how they affect you as you seek to achieve your health and wellness goals.

IDENTIFYING YOUR CORE VALUES

To start the exploration process and get a sense of what your core values are, ask yourself:

- What brings me the most joy?
- What gives my life meaning?
- What makes me come alive?
- What am I truly focused on?

If you can articulate answers to these, you'll likely begin to see a pattern that you can boil down into a single theme.

When considering your core values, it's important to be honest with yourself. While "service to others" may sound good, if it's not core to your sense of self, it really shouldn't make the list. Also note that having more values isn't necessarily better. Ideally, you want to live a life that feels fulfilling and in harmony, meaning you shouldn't feel like your values are pulling you in a million different directions. Now is a great time to start practicing how to listen to your heart to discern what feels most true for you. Although you may find it hard to be specific, just remember that this is an iterative process and that you are already on the right track by thinking about the values that drive you.

If you're having trouble tapping into your core values, here's an exercise to get you started.

(Note: If you're anything like me, then you probably find books that give you "homework" kind of stressful. "What if I don't have the answers? Ummm, she gave me three full pages to write down my answers and I've only written five lines. Ugh, I'm clearly not getting it the way I should." As if someone is going to come around and check your homework at the end of class. Take a deep breath—this isn't about that. This is for you, and you alone.)

STEP ONE: EXPLORE

Recall a moment when you felt perfectly aligned, like yourself, in your element. Write it down.

For example: *When I gave my first health and wellness corporate talk.*

STEP TWO: EXTRACT

List what was important to you about that moment. What made it special? Free-write for a bit to get to the guts of what felt most meaningful to you in the moment you identified. For example:

- Sharing my knowledge and insights to help people.
- Talking about something I really care about and believe is truly important.
- Connecting with the audience and watching them experience relief/aha moments/feelings of hope.
- Being authentic and sharing my experiences and personality without holding back.

STEP THREE: REFLECT

Spend some time reviewing what you wrote. Do you see a pattern? Are there any themes that seem to be coming up? Write down your observations. For example:

- I enjoy being creative.
- I need to feel passionate about where I'm investing my time and energy.
- I love performing.
- Being vulnerable is important to me.
- I thrive when I feel like I'm making a difference.

STEP FOUR: REFINE

Create a list of values based on your findings. There is no right or wrong answer, and your list can change as you tweak and refine further. This is just a starting point to get you thinking about what matters most to you. For example:

- Authenticity
- Vulnerability
- Meaningful work
- Passion
- Connectedness
- Leadership

REFLECT AND REMEMBER

Reflect

Have you been operating based on your own values, or have they been legacy values based on your upbringing, or even more convoluted values based on social media? Do you experience a disconnect between what you feel like you should care about and what you really care about? What feels important to you now?

Remember

1. Values have a major influence on your behavior and determine what you do with your time.

2. When you become consciously aware of your values, you can use them to make more informed decisions about your health and wellness goals instead of just winging it and hoping for good behavior.

3. When considering your own values, it's important to be brutally honest with yourself. Sure, there's a ton of stuff that sounds good, but you need to be straight-up with yourself about what you really care about and why.

3

Surfing the Vortex

YOU MIGHT BE FEELING A little annoyed right now. What does all this have to do with health and wellness? You bought this book to get to the bottom of the whole "when will I finally look and feel as fit as I want to?" issue, and now you're stuck thinking about the bigger picture of your life.

Here's the point: Our values define how we live and what our priorities are. We use them to determine whether life is turning out the way we want it to or not. If you don't know what your evaluation criteria are, how can you even determine whether you're on track or off track? When your values are clear, it's easy to see whether you're living in alignment with them. Once I started to explore my core values, I quickly realized that I was fighting a perfectionist's battle for the ideal body when what I really wanted was to create a foundation of self-love and self-care that would support me throughout my life. Sure, that would involve eating well and working out, but instead of approaching it from a place of self-loathing and criticism, what I actually wanted was to respect my body, fuel it with nourishing food, and challenge it physically so that I could maximize my potential. At my core I craved the ability to support myself through kind words, actions, and love. I wanted to be able to forgive myself if and when I slipped up, and I wanted to anchor myself in the unwavering belief that I was "good enough" *as is*, instead of being someone who constantly needed to be *fixed*.

When it comes to your body, your values impact every aspect of your health and wellness journey. They determine whether you go to the gym and how often, what kind of workouts you do, what kind of diet you're on, and what kinds of drastic measures you do or don't take to get the results you're after.

If you're sick of falling off the wagon time and time again, then you need to clarify your internal "why" to keep your motivational fire going, once and for all.

Yes, the journey is always going to be complicated, but if you can align yourself with your values, you'll be far less likely to veer off track. And even when you do, it'll be a minor detour rather than a full-blown rebound.

I have to warn you, though: Living in alignment is not always easy, particularly when you're living in the #hashtag world. It's no overnight thing. Rather, it's a process. You need to not only define your values but also refine them again and again until they become the yardstick by which you measure your goals, decisions, and actions. It's hard because the #hashtag world can make you feel like you're participating in a never-ending game of tug-of-war, every post you see pushing and pulling you out of alignment.

Even though you know better.

Even though you're committed.

Even though you've done "the work."

It's so easy to get sucked into the vortex, only to find yourself slipping away from who you really are.

But there's so much value in staying aligned.

Clarifying my personal values has helped me make decisions more quickly. I've also found that I regularly feel a greater level of satisfaction with my decisions. It's a daily work in progress, but ever since I committed to living in alignment, there has been a domino effect of goodness in my world.

The cycle looks like this:

- My values have led me to better, faster, and more confident decision-making.
- Stronger and more aligned decisions have increased my satisfaction in life.
- Satisfaction has led me to greater confidence, self-worth, and fulfillment.
- This has further reinforced and strengthened my values.

The overall result has been a much greater sense of ease and flow in my day-to-day life. But trust me, I know it's not easy to switch from where you are now to where you want to go. It took me twenty-five years.

It wasn't until I had checked off all my parents' ticky marks (which I thought were my own) that I realized my life didn't satisfy many of my personal core values, beliefs, and desires. And while I eventually decided to change the game and climb a different mountain altogether, my journey continues. I, too, have to keep refining my personal evaluation criteria and core values, because the #hashtag world keeps me on my toes, tugging me in many directions.

I know it may feel easier to go with the flow and see where the current of life takes you, but the value-finding process is essential to finally getting rid of all the excess noise, mental chatter, wavering, and questioning about your health and wellness goals, happiness, and overall satisfaction in life.

THE *REAL* WORK

Here's my formula for zeroing in on your values: create a Mindset Manifesto. Creating a personal manifesto will not only guide you in setting your wellness goals but also make ongoing decision-making easier. This declaration will capture the essence of what it means to be your "best self " by defining what you truly want and how you intend to live. The purpose of this manifesto is to be a touchstone during the good times and bad, to re-ground you to an articulation of your highest, aspirational self. It's a verbal articulation of the values that matter most to you, which, once articulated, is a binding force that holds you accountable and propels you on your path. It helps you focus on your priorities and serves as a catalyst to move your values into actions.

When you think about your values, you should experience feelings of authenticity and strength. Grab a pen and a pretty notebook (if you're anything like me) or a scrap piece of whatever (if you're anything like my husband) and get started. Iterate and refine until it feels right. Remember, this is real life, not social media.

STEP ONE: WRITE DOWN MINDSET MANIFESTO

Ask yourself: What does wellness mean to me? Think beyond the obvious stuff like diet and exercise and include elements such as your relationships, self-care, personal growth, and social media consumption. Reflect on the values you identified in the previous chapter. What do you want to focus your energy on going forward so that you achieve better inner and outer alignment? Think about these questions as you jot down your ideas:

- What do you like about yourself, your body, and your life as it is now?
- What isn't part of your life now that you wish was?
- What results are you looking to achieve to feel like you're in better harmony?
- What energizes you? When do you feel most alive?
- How will you feel as your best self?

It doesn't matter if you craft a full paragraph statement or if you do a verbal dump. What matters is that you capture the essence of what you really value.

STEP TWO: VISUALIZE IT

Get comfortable, sit in a quiet place, close your eyes, and take a few deep breaths. Inhale deeply for four counts, hold for four counts, and exhale for four counts. Do this several times until you feel like you've really dropped into the present moment.

Now picture yourself in your ideal state of wellness.

- What do you look like?
- What does it feel like?
- What are you doing?
- Where are you spending your time?
- Who are you with?

Picture the details and live in that reality for as long as it feels good.

STEP THREE: REFINE IT

During your visualization, if you find yourself coming up with elements that you didn't include in your Mindset Manifesto, augment your notes. Don't be afraid to reflect on your statement often to make sure it continues to resonate with you. You'll be using this declaration to assess whether your actions are in line with your values, so you want to make sure it's as accurate as it can be.

LIVE BY YOUR VALUES

A word of caution: It's one thing to come up with a manifesto but another thing to actually *live* by your values. That involves focus and commitment. Truly living your values happens during your small, day-to-day decisions (like if you choose to look at Instagram first thing in the morning while still in bed) and your reactions to situations that aren't a part of your "master plan" (like how you choose to handle treats at the office or a spontaneous date night orchestrated by your partner).

We're human beings. It's unrealistic to think that we'll have perfect track records when it comes to aligning with our values. From force of habit to the temptation of immediate gratification, life will often throw us things that can make even the best of us forget our good intentions and act in ways that don't align with our values. However, as with most things in life, alignment improves with practice.

Read your Mindset Manifesto every Sunday before the new week begins. When starting out, you may even want to keep your list handy and read it daily. Take the time to regularly reconnect with what matters to you so you can recommit your focus and attention. Repetition is key. And when you find yourself straying from your vision, approach and analyze the situation with curiosity.

Why did I snooze my alarm instead of going to the gym?

Why did I spend thirty minutes doom scrolling the #hashtag world when I was supposed to be focusing on work?

Why did I eat several tablespoons of peanut butter before going to bed?

Rather than feeling guilty or ashamed, use the experience as a learning opportunity to figure out how you can do better next time. There is no punishment for veering off track. Remember, we're all works in progress.

Speak your values. If your partner, friends, and family are aware of your intentions, there's a greater chance they'll support your desire for change. Now, don't get me wrong, this doesn't mean you have to start posting about your values on social media. The point is that you're striving to live in better alignment rather than putting on a show. So post, or don't post. It's all about doing what *truly* feels right for you.

REFLECT AND REMEMBER

Reflect:

Are you committed to doing things differently this time around? Are you ready for the real work instead of going with the flow, hoping for the best? What kind of mental chatter, wavering, and second-guessing is coming up for you?

Remember

1. Identify your core values ASAP. Doing so will help you zero in on what really matters and shut out the noise—parents, social media, your spouse, whatever.

2. To be certain that you're making the right big and small decisions, you need to know what you're working toward and why. Keep asking yourself and keep refining until it feels right.

3. The values you grew up with may or may not apply to you anymore. That's okay. You must be willing to let go and start fresh. By doing so, you'll be saying "f*ck off" to a lot of useless baggage that's been weighing you down, and you'll lead a happier, lighter life—figuratively and literally.

4

Stop Being an Asshole (to Yourself)

IT WAS A BEAUTIFUL SUNNY day, fresh with possibility. All four of my scheduled alarms went off (5:45, 6, 6:15, 6:30). I scrolled through my Instagram feed as if it were the morning news and then slipped out of bed to get on with the day. I caught a glimpse of myself in the bathroom mirror, and then—like clockwork—the narrative began:

Holy shit, I look tired today. I got enough sleep last night, so is this just what my face looks like now? I swear my under-eye circles are getting darker by the day. Should I switch products again? Who am I kidding? Nothing's going to work; it never does. Okay, forget my face; maybe I'm skinnier today. Nope. Look at my stomach. I shouldn't have eaten so late last night. Oh god, it's only six in the morning and I already feel gross. Maybe it's PMS? Maybe it's pre-PMS. It's not, it's just what my body looks like now. Even if I drop ten pounds, I still won't look fit. God, I'm so negative. I bet everyone else is already up and at 'em, doing all the things I could never do—meditating, journaling, drinking matcha. I bet everyone else is feeling hopeful and positive. I bet everyone else doesn't deal with this shit all the time.

Yup, that used to be me.

Exhausting, am I right?

You've probably had similar thoughts running through your head this past week. Or month. Or year. In fact, you've probably had subtle variations of this harsh narrative about your body, weight, and size on repeat for years. In your voice, in your partner's voice, in the voices of every single person you think is watching you on social media.

- "I can't keep the weight off because I'm just not meant to be skinny."
- "I always fall off the wagon because I can't stay committed."
- "I'm always fighting temptation because I lack discipline."

Does this sound familiar? Mmhmm. I thought so.

Why do we carry these voices around with us? The constant negativity feels excruciating, and yet we still pour salt on our wounds by living in the #hashtag world. Every glam picture, every recipe reel, every before-and-after transformation amplifying our inner pain.

STOP PLAYING TO THE BEAT OF YOUR LIMITING BELIEFS

You may not have recognized your own negative chatter in the past, but I'm sure you've noticed these negative thought patterns in other people. We all have those classic "Debbie

Downer" friends who always feel like they're never going to find love, never going to make enough money, never going to lose weight, or never going to get the promotion.

After listening to your friend's bullshit for years, you get to the point where you just want to shake them and say, "Shut the hell up and do something about it!" But pause for a second. I want you to sit back for a moment and evaluate your own negative thought patterns. I want you to connect with the voices in your head that tell you that you shouldn't get your hopes up too high, that you might be good but so-and-so is better, that you're pretty but not "Instagram pretty," or that you should just be happy with what you have because it's pretty good and frankly the best it will get for you.

You know, the voices that disguise themselves as friendly and helpful. The ones that are there to make sure you don't get too disappointed when you don't get what you want. Sure, when you first tune in, the voices may seem supportive. But are they really? I don't think so. In fact, I suspect that all the gentle, kind reminders in your head are actually pretty mean, covertly insisting that you keep playing to the beat of your limiting beliefs.

Here's how the limiting belief cycle goes:

- **You have a bad experience.** Let's say you attend your first Body Pump class with your coworker only to feel out of place, out of shape, and embarrassed because you can't keep up with the class regulars.

- **You avoid trying it again.** You shy away from the potential for more pain. You begin to casually ignore your coworker's texts and pretend to be injured every time she corners you in the office to set up your next fitness date.

- **If you do try again, you half-ass it.** A group of colleagues is going to Body Pump again because your coworker has made it her mission to make "fitness fun for everyone!" and you don't want to be left out of the group, so you begrudgingly go but put in a solid 3/10 level of effort while you're there. This is so you can point to it and say, "See, it didn't work. I was right."

- **You never get better at the activity.** You double down on the fact that you suck at group fitness.

- **It becomes a self-fulfilling prophecy.** You never try again and therefore never get better at it. Screw Body Pump!

Can you see how clearly this cycle mirrors what most of us go through when it comes to our health and wellness journeys? We do it again and again and again. And let me say, these limiting beliefs don't just impact people who lack confidence. They strike us high-performing, must-be-in-control type A's just as hard.

I spent years of my life at the mercy of my negative self-talk, never feeling smart enough, pretty enough, skinny enough, talented enough, or successful enough:

- "I'll never be seen as beautiful. I get that I'm not ugly, but I'm not actually beautiful."

- "I'm not really smart. I have to study extra hard to get the results I want."

- And, most recently, "I'm not a writer. Who the hell am I to be writing a book?!"

In fact, I wasted an entire year spinning myself in circles about writing a book even though I was the one who decided to take the step in the first place. Nobody forced me. Both the original idea and the decision to execute on that idea were entirely my own. Yet, no matter how hard I tried, I stayed stuck in my head for an entire year. I just couldn't shut out the voices that were constantly saying, "Nothing you have to say is important. It's all been said before. It's basic at best. You're basic at best. What makes you an expert? You're still dealing with all this shit yourself." These voices weren't my own. They were imagined criticisms with a chokehold on me.

So much fear of people coming for me in the comments.

Tearing apart my most vulnerable work.

It was all too much.

When I gave my best friend a watered-down list of my recurring negative thoughts, her exact reaction was, "Holy shit! Sonia, you're a total asshole to yourself. How is all of this judgment and negativity going to help you achieve the things you so badly want to achieve?! Seriously. You're. So. Mean."

The reality is that everybody experiences self-talk throughout the day, whether it's about our bodies, careers, capabilities, intellect, or beauty. Some of our thoughts are positive, but more often our inner narrative is filled with statements that question, judge, and undermine our choices, desires, and self-worth. It happens every time we scroll social media. Every time we compare ourselves to the "perfection" online. Every time we compromise our authenticity for the sake of "likes." Not only does this hurtful narrative have the power to stop us from doing something we truly desire, like when we choose not to wear a sexy dress because we're worried about back fat, but it also perpetuates our fears, limits our potential, stalls our dreams, and forces us into a predetermined future.

So how do you stop the negative chatter and overcome whatever's holding you back from achieving your dreams? First, you need to understand what you really believe and why.

YOUR ENEMIES ARE MAKE-BELIEVE

Beliefs form the foundation of our expectations and determine our actions. They influence 95 percent of the decisions we make and help us better understand ourselves, others, and the world around us. Beliefs aren't facts, but they're often so deeply ingrained in our brains that they can be mistaken for facts, even though they're just conclusions we've drawn based on our experiences, influences, education, and fears.

More specifically, limiting beliefs are the stories we tell ourselves about who we are that hold us back from becoming who we're meant to be. They're the false beliefs that prevent us from pursuing our goals and desires. They're the stories that limit us from reaching our full potential.

They're the reason we sabotage our success.

For years one of my biggest limiting beliefs was that I would never measure up to my big brother, Sanjeev. He was a chronic overachiever. He was a talented pianist and star tennis player. He went to "gifted school" and, as I mentioned earlier, became an engineer *and* a doctor. He was quiet, polite, and an old soul at heart, essentially the exact opposite of everything I was. Everything seemed to come effortlessly to him, which only made me feel worse, and so I pushed extra hard to check off all my parents' ticky marks. It was exhausting.

Chasing academic success.

Chasing notoriety.

Chasing the picture-perfect existence.

We all have past narratives—those stories that fuel us for a long time, like "I'm not as smart as my brother." But at some point, we need to let those go and spend some time creating our own ticky marks for our lives.

Your beliefs may have served you when you were a child, which is why you've hung on to them for so long. For example, my belief that I had to measure up to my brother pushed me to achieve. However, now that you're a fully grown adult, I suspect that many of your beliefs have become legacy beliefs that are a real pain in your ass because they're no longer compatible with your life. Understanding how your beliefs impact your feelings is fundamental, because your beliefs can present you with a false view of reality that exists only in your imagination.

When I look back at my life so far, I can see that there have been several milestones that helped me break free from the mold that I desperately tried to squeeze myself into as a young girl. You've heard a few of them already. But the most liberating moment—the one that served as a final hurdle before I really found my stride—was something much bigger. Something much scarier. Something much more intense.

It was . . . a haircut.

It happened shortly after I graduated from university and started my career, on a Saturday afternoon, while I was visiting Montreal with a group of my friends. We had enjoyed a delicious brunch and were feeling happy and relaxed when we strolled past a fancy French hair salon. I didn't go to Montreal with the intention of cutting my hair; it wasn't even something that had crossed my mind. But there I was, on the old, romantic streets of Montreal, suddenly feeling a desperate pull to take a risk and do something that I had always secretly wanted to do: chop off all my hair.

Let me take a step way back to one of my oldest, deepest legacy beliefs. This belief was so deeply ingrained in my psyche that my parents never had to say a word about it because *they knew* that *I knew* what was expected:

"Indian girls are only considered beautiful if they have luscious long hair."

Growing up as a Sikh girl, I had long hair without ever questioning it. It just was what it was. And, frankly, I loved it because it made me feel kind of like a princess to have thick locks blowing in the wind.

But somewhere along the way, things changed. My blossoming insecurities and harsh self-talk started to attack the loving relationship I once had with my hair. From puberty-induced hair frizz to my desperate desire to keep up with the "cool girls" (who were all suddenly showing up at school with the signature Rachel Green choppy bob), my tender little pre-teen heart started to feel the need to be stylish, beautiful, and cool. My once-beloved long hair had started to make me feel like everyone's ugly-duckling friend—just a bit too unpolished and old-school to effectively blend in with the cool kids.

When it came down to it, there were two conflicting legacy beliefs at play for me:

- Long, virgin hair symbolized my duty to honor my parents and my culture.
- Keeping up with style trends meant I was cool and beautiful and, most importantly, that I fit in.

Growing up, I thought about my hair a lot because it represented the daily dance between my duty to make my parents proud and my desperate desire to take risks and feel free. My ten-, eleven-, and twelve-year-old selves would often sneakily cut inches off my hair to see if I would get caught. In my corporate life, you'd frequently find me pinning my long hair up in a high pony or messy bun, trying to find a creative balance between keeping my parents happy and fitting in as a style-conscious twenty-something starting to find her identity.

Which brings us back to Montreal.

You'd think by this point in my adult life, I would have swiftly moved past the whole fear-of-utterly-disappointing-my-parents thing, but standing outside the salon in Montreal, I found myself making yet another panicky pros and cons list. Was it best to make the bold choice and face their disappointment once again, or to stay stuck and change nothing?

I wanted change. I wanted a new haircut. I knew it would look good. And seriously, it was becoming clear to me just how pathetic it was that I, a twenty-four-year-old adult, was still crippled by the fear of my parents' disapproval, especially about something as superficial as my hair.

For the first time, it was crystal clear to me that something I wanted was right in front of me. So, I took the plunge, and despite feeling nervous, nauseated, and sweaty, I also felt a twinge of pride for jumping into the deep end feet first. There was no going back to the old me, and frankly, my parents were just going to have to deal!

Now here's the supremely stupid part of the story. When I got home, my mom looked at me and said, "Oh wow, your haircut is fantastic. It's so chic and stylish. You look amazing."

*What. In. The. Actual. F*ck.*

Where was the disappointment?

Where were the harsh words?

Where was the godforsaken look?

I felt delirious at first, like I had made up this huge narrative about my parents that wasn't even true. Had I completely fabricated the parental shackles that I felt had been holding me back for so long?

No, I didn't make it all up. But I *was* allowing limiting beliefs, instead of reality, to dictate my feelings and actions. As an adult, I had unknowingly allowed my thoughts to hold me back, and when I witnessed my mom's reaction, I could clearly see that I was the one who had placed the imaginary shackles on myself.

DISMANTLE YOUR LIMITING BELIEFS

It feels ridiculous to say out loud that something as small as a haircut had such a tremendous impact on my life, but I'll say it anyway. It's the truth. In a very roundabout sort of way, cutting off my hair taught me that standing out was something I wanted and that choosing the road less traveled, but the one that I was called to, made me feel more like myself than anything ever had before. By confronting my limiting beliefs, breaking through my old stories, and choosing a different path, I found . . . freedom.

Moral of the story? Freedom comes when we understand that at the root of all of our behaviors is a set of beliefs. We must get to know them. Befriend them. Make peace with them. And then gently drop the ones that no longer serve us. Coming face to face with our inner narrative takes courage, but when we do this work, we open ourselves up to new possibilities. It's a work in progress that I practice every day.

I practice shutting out the noise.

I practice tuning in to which voices are taking the lead in my head.

I practice staying anchored to my gut because without solid footing, it's just too easy for me to get sucked into the vortex.

Here's the deal: You hold on to beliefs regardless of whether or not they serve you in the present moment because they provide you with a sense of certainty and peace of mind. Human beings *love* certainty and peace of mind. Beliefs can reduce stress, anxiety, and fear. The problem is that you (and your life) keep changing, but your beliefs remain constant, which causes you to feel stuck. When your beliefs aren't aligned with your goals and objectives, you essentially feel stranded, unfulfilled, and miserable.

Your beliefs stay with you even if they no longer serve you well.

You want to lose weight? You want to be strong? You want to feel beautiful? I hate to say it, but those things can't happen if you don't shut out the external noise and clarify how your belief system is failing to align with your goals and objectives.

If you think you're immune to limiting beliefs, just know that we all carry these success-limiting mantras around with us. They impact:

- **The labels you give yourself.** "I'm always going to be kind of chunky." "I'm too much of a foodie to eat healthy." "I'm not as genetically blessed as those fit girls at the gym."

- **The limitations you put on yourself.** "I can't sign up for the gym; I won't fit in." "I can't go to that group fitness class; I'm too much of an amateur." "I can't do weekly meal prep; I'm not that hardcore."

- **The expectations you have for yourself.** "I'll never actually lose weight." "I'll always be unhappy with my body; that'll never change." "I'll never look good naked."

Your belief system serves as the lens through which you perceive the world, and when you're wearing murky gray glasses every day, you sure as hell can expect to feel undeserving and unhappy. Limiting beliefs prevent you from changing, keep you blind to opportunities in your path, and prevent you from accepting gifts from the Universe. When you believe disappointment is a foregone conclusion, you shun risk, retreat to your comfort zone, and operate on autopilot to prevent losing control or getting hurt.

The result?

Your body remains the same.

The way you feel about your body remains the same.

And the pain is real.

It doesn't matter where your limiting beliefs originated. What matters is that you take some time to reflect on them, understand how limiting beliefs are stopping you from achieving your health and wellness goals, and dismantle them.

REFLECT AND REMEMBER

Reflect

How can you identify your limiting beliefs and catch them as they come into play? Do you feel like you're ready to dissect your negative chatter so that you can discern fact from fiction? In doing so, you'll be able to use logic and reasoning to squash your limiting beliefs and push past your fears.

Remember

1. Beliefs form the foundation of your expectations and dictate your decisions and your actions.

2. Limiting beliefs don't just impact people who lack confidence. Whether or not you realize it, you experience constant self-talk throughout the day, and often, it's extremely negative.

3. Your beliefs stay with you, even if they no longer serve you well. You must clarify how your belief system is failing to align with your objectives to achieve your health and wellness goals.

5

Changing Your Narrative

YOUR PERSONAL PATTERNS MAY LOOK different from mine, but however your limiting beliefs are manifesting themselves, one thing is for certain: They are holding you back from achieving your goals. They are preventing you from taking crucial steps to change how you look and how you feel about your body, your self-worth, and your satisfaction in life. And at the most basic, day-to-day level, they're driving you to engage in behaviors that are sabotaging your progress and preventing you from following through with the lifestyle choices needed to achieve your health and wellness goals.

Having limiting beliefs about your body seems to be what society expects. Heck, it's become the norm for us to talk shit about our love handles and muffin tops. Who actually goes around saying, "I think I look amazing. No, seriously, I'm so proud of my ass!" Nobody. Why? Because being self-deprecating is considered a good trait. We don't like people who think they're better than us. We don't like people who come off as conceited. We like people who feel bad about themselves because they make us feel like it's okay for us to feel bad about ourselves, too. As long as people straddle that perfect line between hating themselves and loving themselves, we feel right at home.

However, it's important to recognize that if you've got limiting beliefs about your body, those beliefs are likely also rearing their ugly heads in various other facets of your life:

- **Career.** "What's the point in applying for this job? I probably won't get it anyway. Even if I do get the job, I probably won't stack up against everyone who already works there."

- **Love.** "There's no point in trying to put myself out there because I'm not what they're looking for." "Why should I leave this relationship when there's nothing better out there for me?"

- **Lifestyle.** "Why bother trying to start working out when I'm not going to be able to keep up with it? I can't get organized, meal prep, and pack my meals."

- **Motherhood.** "She's the type who can do it all, but I'm not." "I'm not structured enough, disciplined enough, affectionate enough."

If you can't already see it, let me spell it out for you: all this negativity is causing you to give up on some very attainable goals in your life. So, what do you do with this fact? How do you move forward?

IT'S TIME TO GET UNSTUCK

I know this is likely starting to feel a bit heavy right now, so let me share some good news: you are not just some asshole who likes to say mean, assholey things about yourself to yourself.

Let me repeat: you are not inherently an asshole.

Each limiting belief you hold serves a purpose. At their core, these beliefs are just trying to protect you from pain. They may not make any real sense and may be completely impractical, but each limiting belief you hold really does have good intentions. Those intentions are just totally misguided because while your beliefs may protect you from short-term pain, they unfortunately lead to long-term pain.

I know you know better. We all do. But even though you know better, just like I did, separating yourself from a twenty-plus-year narrative that you've come to deeply believe as your truth is easier said than done. Most of us aren't in tune yet, and even those of us who are still need to fine-tune further.

Each time we check our phones.

Each time we post a picture.

Each time we respond to a comment.

We need to fine-tune so intensely that we can catch and release each and every limiting belief we hold about ourselves, others, and the world around us until we can change what we believe and the way we talk to ourselves.

Does anybody want to wake up to the negativity that's been simmering beneath the surface? No, not really. But I promise all this effort will be worth it. If you're sick of feeling like you're stuck, if you're tired of feeling like you're always facing the same challenges, if you're done with feeling like you can't achieve your goals, then abolishing your limiting beliefs is the only way to break the cycle.

BE YOUR OWN HYPE WOMAN

One of the most valuable practices you can do for yourself when working toward shifting your perspective and becoming your own cheerleader is operate with compassion.

Imagine you're engaging with a close friend or maybe even your child, niece, or nephew; think of someone you'd want to really nurture and support. How would you speak to them if they were sharing their negative thoughts and fears with you? What would you say to guide them through the situation? I bet you'd listen attentively, empathize, and try to show them the way forward with genuine support. You'd shine a light on all the good they bring to the table, you'd offer them different perspectives to show them the right path, and you'd remind them not to be too hard on themselves.

How would your life change if you were your own biggest fan?

How would it change the way you talk to yourself?

The choices you make?

The way you walk in the world?

I know, this advice sounds a little fluffy, like a bit of self-help bullshit. But one of the most important things I've learned throughout my life is this: you are the one constant in your life, and when you can show up for yourself (without being an asshole to yourself), your life gets a whole lot better. All the harsh self-talk is not only exhausting to listen to all day long, but also really ineffective in getting us the results we want. In fact, it often sets us back exponentially.

I used to be an incredibly harsh frenemy to myself. For years, my daily dialogue looked something like this: "Don't get your hopes up; you'll probably never look the way you want to. It's just unrealistic, given your genetically thick arms and flat butt. Keep trying, sure, but you won't be happy until you look the way you want to . . . and that's probably not going to happen."

My inner dialogue was so destructive largely because I feared being average, although I criticized myself daily for being nothing special. I desperately wanted to prove my worth to my loved ones and the world, although the voice in my head told me I would never shine in their eyes. I craved success and validation to feel good enough, and even when I was met with success, it never felt fulfilling or big enough. I deeply wanted to feel beautiful, although I quietly called myself ugly and picked apart all the tiny flaws I saw.

I feel sorry for that version of who I was. It hurts me to think I wasted so much of my life hating myself, when instead I could have been using all that energy to build up my self-esteem and self-worth. But looking back on my old dialogues also makes me feel thankful for how far I've come and shows me that it really has been an incredible journey of learning and growing.

Today my inner dialogue looks drastically different.

A few months ago, when I felt exhausted, overwhelmed, and uninspired for so many reasons, I felt a strong pull to take a break from social media. Oddly enough, this is often considered a giant risk when you're supposedly an "influencer." Where did this desire come from? When I took the time to unpack it, I realized that I was back in the cycle of limiting beliefs. "You're not good enough. Your content is shittier than other influencers. People say they want authenticity, but they really want perfect people and you're anything but perfect."

The voice went on and on. But instead of succumbing to it, I really stepped up with care and compassion and tried to use what I had learned over the years: *talk to yourself like you would talk to your best friend.*

I evaluated my feelings without judgment: I felt misaligned. I felt burnt out. I felt like shutting down. The way that I had been showing up online wasn't working for me anymore.

I took the time to understand my needs: I needed to take a step back to actually reconnect and nurture myself. I needed a break from the hamster wheel of online performance. I needed a shift in priorities to cultivate better long-term balance.

I took action without hesitation: I gave myself a much-needed hiatus from social media and felt a sense of calm, knowing that I had approached myself with understanding, compassion, and respect. I felt inspired and empowered, and when I resurfaced on social media, I felt like I was back in the driver's seat of my life, both online and offline.

Are you ready to shift the way you relate and speak to yourself?

GET CURIOUS

To start to shift how you talk to yourself, you need to do a little detective work. For a few days, pay close attention to your inner dialogue:

- What is your tone? What is the emotion behind your tone?
- Are you angry more often than not?

- Are you constantly blaming others? Are you constantly blaming yourself?
- Does this energy extend to the world around you?
- Do you feel compassion and empathy toward others?
- Do you feel compassion toward yourself?

Let's take this exploration further.

LIMITING BELIEFS, AN EXERCISE

Think back to an accomplishment that you're proud of and become aware of your emotions and physical response to that memory. Does your chest feel lighter when you think back to that moment? Do your shoulders drop? Do you feel the urge to smile?

Now think about a current goal or dream. How do you feel when you think about it? Chances are, your first mental, emotional, and physical reactions are positive.

You may feel a little rush.

You may feel the urge to smile.

You may feel excited.

Then, depending on how severe your limiting beliefs are, you'll likely begin to feel worse. You may experience a slight tightness in your body or even a hint of nausea. You may start to feel a light sweat in your palms or your shoulders rising to your ears. Your breath may begin to shorten ever so slightly. This is your subconscious mind trying to convince you that what you're dreaming about is dangerous and that you shouldn't do it. *Et voilà*, your limiting beliefs are firing up to get you to stay put!

Take note. Write down the feelings. Capture the sensations. Sit with them for a bit. Repeat this process again for your top five current desires.

Try to name your limiting beliefs. Don't stress about whether you're getting the words right, just focus on what you feel like they represent to you. Nobody is going to see this list, so give yourself permission to get a little raw and dirty here. For example:

- I'm too old or too young.
- I'm too fat or too skinny, too tall or too short.
- I'm never going to look like the people I follow online.
- I'm not smart enough.
- I'm too far behind everyone else to catch up.
- I'm not connected enough.
- I'm never going to be able to achieve my goals.
- I can't start. I'm not ready.

Once you've got your list, it's time to practice letting go of your limiting beliefs and start empowering yourself with positive ones.

Look at the list of your limiting beliefs. Let's say one of your beliefs is "I can't go to the gym." Question it.

Throw doubt on it.

Why can't I go to the gym? Just because I was too uncomfortable last time doesn't mean I won't feel differently this time. Lots of people go to the gym regardless of how fit they are.

Consider the consequences of your limiting beliefs. What happens if things don't change?

I'll have a harder time achieving my fitness goals. I won't be able to lose weight the way I want to. I'll continue to feel unhealthy and out of shape.

Create new, positive, empowering beliefs to adopt instead. What would someone who wants to accomplish your goals believe about themselves?

I'm not the same person as I was back then. I can set small, attainable goals so that I gain momentum. I can ease into it with a friend.

Firmly decide that you are going to change. Tear up your list of limiting beliefs. Burn it. Bury it. Let that shit go. Remember, your limiting beliefs run deep. You must be committed, motivated, and determined to change the narrative. Create some new, positive belief statements:

- I'm doing this for me.
- I've committed to a gym schedule.
- I'm not starting again; I'm building on experience.

Make room for these new beliefs in your life. Say them frequently and work hard to change your habits to align with your new version of reality. Set boundaries. Take space from the #hashtag world when it causes your limiting beliefs to flare up so that you're not being pushed and pulled away from your new, empowering beliefs. Take space from all that doesn't serve the direction you're moving in, because you deserve some breathing room. Take action frequently until it starts to feel more comfortable. The point of all this is to gently bring yourself face to face with the narrative that's holding you back. It's not meant to be grueling. It's not punishment.

Don't let your limiting beliefs about yourself and your body rule your life. You are so much more than your body, and bringing doubt and negativity into the mix not only creates unnecessary stress but also robs you of joy.

REFLECT AND REMEMBER

Reflect

Are you ready to clarify your true intentions in order to eliminate the noise and distractions that have been getting in your way? Once you know what's preventing you from hitting your stride, you'll be able to address those blocks and begin to hone in on your health and wellness goals while sidestepping the usual self-sabotaging on-again, off-again bullshit.

Remember

1. Whether or not you believe it, you've got negative chatter going on in your mind that's holding you back from achieving your goals. There are some harsh limiting beliefs driving these cruel thoughts, and they need to be cleared away.

2. To achieve long-term results, you need to shift two key elements: your relationship with yourself and your belief system. You do this by discerning fact from fiction. It's not a quick fix, but all it really takes is a bit of judgment-free detective work and curiosity about your mental chatter.

3. Roadblocks disappear once you can identify where your fear is limiting you. Most of our fears come from limiting beliefs, and once we clear them, we're empowered to feel great about our actions, progress, and results.

6

Where Do the Happy People Live?

IN TODAY'S INSTA-LIVING WORLD, IT'S easy to feel like perfection is no longer an impossible standard. When you scroll through your social media feed, how often do you see anything but perfectly curated images of perfect relationships, perfect bodies, perfect faces, and perfect success stories?

We even see just enough "perfect imperfection" to make us feel like, "Yes, that person's version of imperfect is #goals— not too raw, not too messy, *just enough* to be semi-relatable." Sure, somewhere in our rational minds we know better. We know that there's no such thing as perfect, but the illusion of perfect can mess with the best of us.

The pursuit of perfection made me feel like shit for years. It polluted my thoughts, overshadowed my logic, and robbed me of so many simple pleasures. I knew all the things, like:

- "You don't have to be perfect to be amazing."
- "There is no perfection, only beautiful versions of brokenness."
- "You were born to be real, not perfect."

Yet perfectionism wove its way in and out of every nook and cranny in my life. It led me to people-pleasing for decades. It reared its head in academics from middle school till the end of my MBA. It colored all of my early career choices. It sparked the onset of my disordered eating habits and intense exercise regimen. It led to my all-or-nothing "hamster wheel" approach to health and wellness. Most importantly, and painfully, it led to a mindset that was devoid of balance, compassion, and joy. Did I see any of this at the time? No, of course not. I was living the only way I knew how.

I couldn't see how unhappy I was.

I couldn't see that I was caught in a failure loop caused by self-sabotage.

I couldn't see that I fluctuated from feeling totally numb to feeling incredibly critical and cruel toward myself.

Spoiler alert: Until I did. And then my whole life changed.

RELAX YOUR HANDS ON THE WHEEL

In my experience, perfectionism is the pursuit of ultimate control. It's the way we (try to) control outcomes. It's the way we (try to) control how people perceive us. It's the way we (try to) control how people react to us.

Control. We love it. We chase it because we feel like we *really* need it.

But you know as well as I do that we can't control most things outside of ourselves. Life just isn't set up for perfection, and never have I learned that more than during my struggles with fertility.

I was thirty years old. By science standards and brown-parent standards alike, it was time for me to have a baby. I had been married for almost five years, and I could only delay motherhood for so much longer without having to get defensive about it. I knew I wanted to have kids, and I figured I had finally hit a phase in my career when I could take some time to have a baby, so I decided to do what I do best: make an aggressive plan.

I started by mapping out my timeline, identifying the ideal months for me to pop out this kid based on a variety of factors such as the weather, my husband's residency schedule, seasonal media patterns, and more. I then moved on to the research phase. I knew how the birds and the bees worked, of course, but there had to be some sort of formula I could follow for maximum efficiency. I needed to become a fertility specialist via Google:

- Do you need to prop your legs up after sex?
- How many days a month do you actually ovulate?
- Do hot tubs really kill sperm?

Then I bought the ovulation kits—first the basic sticks, then the hardcore minicomputer because I obviously didn't want to waste time shooting in the dark. In hindsight, that was absolutely ridiculous. I should have insisted that we have all kinds of fun shooting in the dark for a while. Why did I make getting pregnant into some kind of homework? I wanted results, like I always do—immediate results. I wanted to get pregnant now so that I could "move on to the next phase." I wanted to conquer pregnancy the way I always forced myself to conquer phases.

The Universe had other plans.

I got off the pill, but after a few months I still had no period. It doesn't take a rocket scientist to know that things probably aren't functioning the way they should be in the fertility department if you're not getting a period. I tried not to panic, but I started worrying about what was going on with my insides. You spend so much of your life trying not to get pregnant that rarely do you stop and think, "Oh shit, maybe all this prevention is unnecessary. Maybe I'm barren." You always think that when you want to get pregnant, it will just kind of happen, like in the movies. Bollywood brown girl and brown guy have sex one time on their wedding night and *bam!*

Here's the reality: I had been so busy running hard and running fast that I hadn't stopped to do a real self-check in a long time. I was in such "doing mode" that I didn't ever slow down to make sure that I was really taking care of myself. Yes, I was eating enough to grow and sustain muscle. Yes, I was working out the "right way." Yes, I was in the best shape of my life. But was I really feeling good? Did I have energy? Did I feel like a well-oiled machine? If you had asked me at the time, my answer would have been, "Oh, hell yes, I've never felt better." In hindsight, I think I was just doped up on endorphins and my go-get-'em attitude more than anything. My body wasn't working according to the manual, and something was clearly wrong. It had been only four months, not long enough for me to really start panicking out loud, but I knew something wasn't right, and I wanted to resolve the problem ASAP.

I started seeing an acupuncturist who specialized in fertility. I also switched my research from the mechanics of getting pregnant to the mechanics of repairing an infertile body. I layered in all the healthy goodness I could get my hands on, from green smoothies to steel-cut oats to avocado, coconut oil, almonds, and legumes. I even got saucy and incorporated superfoods like spirulina, goji berries, and ashwagandha. I layered in vitamins, I layered in rest days, I layered in tactics to rebalance my hormones, and slowly it seemed like my body was starting to respond. After a couple months of acupuncture and a focused diet, I turned a corner and finally got a period. It was irregular at best, but it had started to come, and I had a glimmer of hope.

Throughout all this, I was scared and embarrassed. Here I was, a supposed health and wellness expert, with a body that couldn't do the one thing it's technically designed to do. I had conquered the external piece of my physique, but had I really mastered anything if I wasn't even aware of and in tune with my internal health? Had I really mastered anything if I was coming up against one of the biggest roadblocks life can throw you? I had an existential crisis. Again.

On one hand, I was scared that maybe I would never get the chance to be a mother. When you start to confront the idea that you might not actually get something, that's often when you realize how badly you want it. On the other hand, I was scared that maybe there was something medically wrong with me. I was used to controlling every aspect of my life. I had been able to apply brute force to anything and it had always worked. But I couldn't do it this time.

Then my doctor told me that my "big" fertility problem was that I had what she called "sss." Skinny successful syndrome—a condition where perfectionist people (usually women) put so much physical and mental stress on themselves that their hormone levels get out of whack and fertility is compromised. That bombshell really made me question who I am. I always knew that balance wasn't my forte, but this was yet another, rather harsh, wake-up call from the Universe.

I couldn't keep pushing myself so hard.

From cycle monitoring, we moved on to hormone pills, self-administered injections, and ultimately intrauterine insemination, which led to my first baby. My time at the fertility clinic feels like a long chapter of my life when I look back at it, but in reality, it wasn't long at all. Within half a year, I had successfully gotten pregnant and was on to the next challenge: the pregnancy itself. I was scared shitless. Scared that I had somehow tricked my body into getting pregnant via the shots and the pills and the turkey basting when it didn't actually have the capacity to *be* pregnant.

I worried about miscarrying every day.

I worried about losing the baby during labor.

I worried about everything all the time because I was scared my body was still not functioning the way it needed to in order to be a safe home for a baby.

The only thing I could do to pacify myself was focus even more on my well-being. I made every effort to connect with my body, to listen to what it was telling me, and to understand what I needed to do with the messages. I ate for health, I worked out for health, and I rested for health. And while it was scary at first, I slowly started to feel like I could trust my body in a way that I never really thought about before. Eventually, something clicked, and I registered that I couldn't orchestrate the perfect fertility outcome or control how my body behaved inside, just like I could never craft the perfect body outside. I released my need to be in complete control.

This shift led to some sweet relief. It was like a weight was slowly being lifted off, knowing that if it wasn't possible for me to control everything, then I also didn't have to feel responsible for every outcome all the time. Sometimes I could just drop my shoulders and stop the over-thinking. Sometimes I could just relax and enjoy the ride.

LEARN TO ENJOY THE RIDE

If you look up "perfectionism" in the dictionary, you'll find something like:

> Perfectionism: (adj.) striving for flawlessness and setting excessively high performance standards accompanied by overly critical self-evaluations and concerns regarding others' evaluations.[1]

Ugh. I'm cringing as I write. That definition brings me right back to who I used to be (. . . and sometimes still am, if I'm not vigilant). I'll be the first to admit, perfectionism is a messy, tough battle to fight.

So why do so many of us struggle with perfectionist tendencies? For starters, the pursuit of perfection is not only deeply ingrained in us as individuals but also rampant in our societal narrative. From our earliest days, our parents drive home the need for perfect obedience and discipline. As we grow older, we come up against expectations around achieving perfect grades, getting admitted into top-tier schools, and securing successful career paths straight out of university. While all this is going on, we're also bombarded with images of perfect faces and perfect bodies and perfect luxuries and perfect relationships in traditional and social media.

It's no wonder that so many of us deeply fear being considered mediocre. As a culture, we also recognize and reward perfectionists for their insistence on setting high standards and their relentless drive to meet those standards. The message is reinforced from all sides: perfect is better.

But life isn't perfect. Remember: perfectionism is not the skill we need to master. Instead, we must focus on mastering resilience, progress, growth, patience, and acceptance. Learning to embrace my imperfection is what has allowed me to continue living in the #hashtag world without feeling like I'm getting sucked into the vortex. It's what has connected me with so many others. It's what has led me to more meaningful interactions and relationships, both online and in the real world. Perfection is incredibly isolating, but the realness of imperfection is what connects us all.

THERE IS NO "END DESTINATION"

When we're raised to believe that perfect is not only possible but expected, something strange begins to happen: "Perfect" as a destination ceases to exist altogether. It merely becomes a mirage in the distance, a never-ending quest that drives us endlessly.

By pursuing unrealistic ideals and ever-evolving goals, we lose sight of who we really are. We become absorbed with end results and fail to take pleasure in the journey. We suffer when we're not achieving perfect track records and often experience incredibly negative self-talk. Despite all this, we can, and often do, conquer some pretty substantial wins, like losing those stubborn ten pounds or getting lean enough to see ab definition. The problem is that even when we do conquer our goals, we feel like we're thriving for only a brief moment. We feel great as long as we get praise and attention and admiration from others and then . . . it's gone. Why does the success feel so fleeting? It's partly because we rely on external sources to validate our worth and partly because we have a deep-seated need to constantly outdo ourselves. Remember those shape-shifting goals we talked about? Without positive feedback and the feeling of an uphill battle, we often fail to feel glory.

Perfectionism equals perpetual dissatisfaction.

The wins are never enough.

REFLECT AND REMEMBER

Reflect

Are you being held hostage by perfectionist tendencies? What resistance comes up for you when you think of yourself as a "perfectionist"?

Remember

1. To strive for perfection is exactly that: the vigorous struggle to become flawless. But the thing is, flawlessness isn't human.

2. You simply can't avoid experiencing the ups and downs that come along with any health and wellness journey, or life in general, for that matter. What you can do, however, is strive to cope better with the ebbs and flows.

3. Perfectionism twists and manipulates the way you think about all aspects of your life. It keeps you striving for impossible standards and leaves you feeling empty, defeated, and inferior when you can't keep up.

7

A Body You Love, a Life You Hate

I USED TO BELIEVE THAT my perfectionist tendencies kept me going. I was like the Energizer Bunny: I could go longer and harder and faster than anyone else around. If you wanted a job done and done perfectly, then I was your girl. When it came to my body, my very aggressive desire to be thinner, leaner, and fitter kept me going. In my mind, if I wasn't progressing toward the perfect body, then I was failing.

I would turn myself into body parts rather than seeing myself as a whole person. Without realizing it, I would break my body down into "areas of focus" to keep myself driven and to keep tackling the next piece of the puzzle.

"All I want is a flat stomach. Then I'll feel good" would soon turn into . . .

"Anyone can have a flat stomach. I need a rounder and firmer butt to really look good," which would soon turn into . . .

"Anyone can have the butt, but when I have definition in my shoulders, then I'll really look fit."

It felt natural to expect more of myself and push myself harder than others. It felt natural to have to struggle for what I wanted. It felt natural to have to *earn* the likes and comments online.

But could I live up to my own ridiculous standards? Nope. I really couldn't.

I was on a roller coaster that never stopped, never made me happy, and never fulfilled me as a human being.

IT'S ALL RUINED

I never *willingly* slowed down.

The intense climate I had created for myself played out in all-or-nothing ways, and as soon as I wavered or experienced a setback, I considered my perfect track record to be ruined.

Sound familiar? (Don't lie to me.)

You're about to kick off a new diet for the week. It's Monday. You've stocked your fridge with healthy meals, you've prepped lunches for the next few days, and you've made an entire workout schedule. After downing a green smoothie, you head into the office feeling determined and in control, and that's when the news breaks: it's somebody's birthday.

And we all know birthdays equal cupcakes.

You feel a little anxious, but you tell yourself, "Nah, I'll be okay. I'm just going to avoid them altogether; I don't even like buttercream." Then a cupcake is hand-delivered to your desk by the birthday girl herself, and she patiently stands in front of you, waiting to do a cupcake-cheers. You can't be an ass-hole and say, "No, I'm good. I care about my diet more than your birth" (although let's be real, you do), so you eat half a cupcake (*God, the icing is delish*) and remind yourself to cut back on lunch.

When you get home at the end of the day, you're famished, and your dry salmon and bland steamed broccoli just aren't cutting it. You add some salad to the mix because when has salad ever hurt anybody, right? And then a few berries for dessert. And then a full handful of berries on top of that. But you're still not satisfied so you go for the healthy fat, something to really soothe your soul, the good stuff—the almond butter. First a tiny little teaspoon, then you're downing several non-serving-size spoonfuls, and that's when the panic sets in.

"Oh shit, I'm way over my daily caloric limit for today."

"Okay, it's no big deal; I guess I technically ate a lot of food, but it was all healthy."

"No, it wasn't. Remember the cupcake? Shit. I knew I should have just said no. Why did I do this to myself? It's fine, I'll start again tomorrow . . . clean slate."

"But tomorrow is Tuesday. Who starts on a Tuesday? Eww. That's practically basically begging for failure. This whole week is ruined. Let me just start again with a clean slate next week. Ugh, *why* did I eat the stupid cupcake!"

And so, the week is ruined. Maybe even the month, depending on how far into the month you are. (Because if you're anything like me, there's always a creative way to rationalize when to start again based on when the first day of the next month is.)

CAN'T STOP, WON'T STOP

Sometimes we make it past that first week. However, even when we do *temporarily* end up with a body we love, we often also end up with a life we kind of hate. The amount of time, effort, and obsession required to inch closer to the perfect body feels great at first, but it becomes truly soul-sucking after a while. With enough effort, you *can* control the way you look, as I did through obsessive eating and exercise addiction. But let's be real, until you receive that acknowledgment and recognition for your visible effects, you don't really feel like you've achieved anything. The problem is that you can't control the feedback you receive from others, and when you live for all that external praise to validate your existence, your self-esteem and self-worth take some seriously tough punches.

Whenever I give a talk about health and wellness and get to perfectionist narratives, I get enthusiastic head nods and nervous giggles from the audience. Most people feel a deep sense of relief when someone points out just how hard we're all making this journey for ourselves. The amount of energy required to pursue perfection is exhausting, and it requires us to behave in a way that is totally contradictory to our biological and psychological programming.

Let me ask you: Are you only this hard on yourself when it comes to your body? Or are you constantly trying to one-up yourself in all aspects of your life? Do you find yourself taking the all-or-nothing approach more often than not? Are you always battling the "when I get there, I'll be happy" narrative? Do you find yourself putting things off because it isn't the right time or because you're not ready?

Here's the reality of the situation: Most perfectionist tendencies don't start and stop in the health and wellness department. They're easy to see when it comes to how you feel about your body, but if you're anything like I used to be (and sometimes still am), this perfectionist stuff is bleeding into all areas of your life.

I realized something important when I started to identify my own symptoms of perfectionism: Perfectionism doesn't have to reach torturous levels to be destructive. Even casual perfectionists who don't think of themselves as perfectionists at all (yes, I'm talking to *you*) can experience the negative side effects of their unwavering pursuit of excellence.

Here are five signs that perfectionism might be at play in your life:

1. **You know your perspective hurts you.** You live by the credo "I achieve, therefore I am," and while you know this isn't healthy, you consider it just a cost of success. You go to great lengths to avoid being average and believe that you won't gain without pain. You know that your relentless standards are unreasonable and stress-inducing, but you believe that they fuel your productivity and excellence.

2. **You procrastinate.** You wait a long time for the moment to be "right" to work on your goals. You start only when you feel totally ready to do your best work, and unfortunately, this "readiness" rarely comes. Despite your intense desire to succeed, you're deeply familiar with excessive procrastination.

3. **You take pleasure in others' failure.** You judge everyone—your friends, your family, the "randos" on the street, everyone in the #hashtag world. You spend time and energy comparing

yourself to others, and you often feel deep (secret) relief when someone experiences a setback or challenge.

4. **You fear failure.** You struggle with black-and-white thinking: you're a success one moment and a failure the next based on your latest accomplishment or setback. You take on a new project only if you believe you'll succeed, and when you aren't turning minor setbacks into major incidents, then you're avoiding playing the game at all.

5. **You can always "aim higher."** You always feel like you could, and should, do more. You focus on what you haven't accomplished yet, which fuels the urge to constantly outdo yourself. You're not happy unless you're on your way to a higher, bigger goal, and you're rarely content with the status quo.[2]

So much negativity.
So harsh.
So painful.

BREAKING DOWN PERFECTIONISM

The great irony of perfectionism is that while it's character-ized by an intense drive to succeed, it's actually propelled by the total fear of failure. It's not that we're actually trying to be "perfect," but rather that we're desperately trying to avoid being "not good enough."

By shunning any risk of failure and deliberately modify-ing our behaviors and habits to match what we think others expect, we detach from our core values.

We feel misaligned.

We feel disconnected from our authentic selves.

We feel stuck.

Here's the deal: Demanding perfection from yourself can only take you so far, and at some point, you will fail. It has to happen. It's a part of life, and it's a part of any health and wellness journey. Perfectionism twists and manipulates the way that you think about food, your body, and yourself, and ultimately, you just can't keep up.

Perfectionist tendencies impact your relationship:

- **With food.** You engage in unnatural eating patterns. You starve yourself when you're hungry. You avoid certain social situations. You refuse to eat anything that isn't "clean."

- **With your body.** You have unrealistic expectations of what you should look like. You engage in constant analysis and comparison. You focus on the superficial. You engage in excessive exercise.

- **With yourself.** You have a deep-seated feeling that you aren't worthy of love because you can't achieve a certain look. If you do achieve your desired look, you become trapped by the fear that people will stop paying attention to you if you fail to maintain it.

My addiction to body perfection was full-blown by the time I was a teenager. Despite being a small-to-medium-sized girl, I was on a desperate quest to lean down.

I wanted to *look* thin.

I wanted to *feel* thin.

I wanted to *be* thin.

And so what was my solution? To stop eating altogether. I knew I'd have to eat dinner every day at home or my parents would know something was up. But when I was at school, I literally ate nothing. I drank water, I chewed a lot of gum, and if I really got hungry, sometimes I'd break the rules and allow myself to eat some saltine crackers. I don't understand how I did it; I wasn't swayed by temptation in the least. Watching people eat didn't bother me at all. I was kind of robotic about it, and to this day I find it hard to believe that I could just shut off the hunger part of my brain.

Did I lose weight? You bet.

Did I love it? Sure did.

My clothes started to feel looser and then slowly, they started to hang off me. I felt incredible. In fact, the looser my clothes fit, the better I felt. I remember how confident and proud my inner narrative had become. I remember how much I loved the attention I got from everyone asking me how I lost weight and saying I "looked so good."

I didn't feel average anymore.

I didn't feel like I wasn't good enough anymore.

I felt successful again.

My disordered eating continued for about a year, at which point I decided to kick things up a notch. Somewhere along the way I concluded that just being skinny wasn't good enough. Being skinny was amateur. It was easy. Heck, a lot of people were born skinny, so what was the accomplishment in that? I needed to be skinny *and* fit, like the girls in the magazines.

That was hot.

That was above average.

That was the new goal.

And so, I began going to the gym every day to do ninety minutes of cardio between the stair climber, treadmill, and elliptical. How I thought that cardio would lead me to have abs and muscle definition is beyond me, but there I was, like so many others, on the hamster wheel of weight loss.

Except that I was running on fumes, and you can only run on empty for so long before you finally burn out. That's exactly what happened. I started to feel tired, sluggish, and fatigued. Most of all, I started to have intense cravings. After exercising willpower for so long and fighting the voices in my head day in and day out, I finally caved and started eating again. Just a little at first, but then it snowballed into a full-on rebound when I went off to university.

PROGRESS OVER PERFECTION

The fact of the matter is this: when you put so much pressure on yourself to achieve perfect track records and perfect scenarios and perfect outcomes, you actually rob yourself of success. When perfectionism is driving you, there's just no way to get out of the vortex. Rather than trying to control every aspect of your life, maybe it's time to pivot your focus and think about achievement in a different way. Instead of pushing yourself impossibly hard and demanding growth through the mastery of perfection, maybe you begin learning to trust and surrender. Maybe you let go of your need for control.

What if you were to embrace the ups and downs of your health and wellness journey (which are inevitable, by the way) and choose to see them as opportunities to learn something new about yourself?

What if you were to build yourself a life full of activities and pursuits that make you feel great instead of doing everything you think the #hashtag world wants you to do?

What if you were to give yourself space beyond all the external pressure to hear what ignites your soul?

You can. It just takes time, understanding, patience, and the commitment to recognize and develop your self-worth.

I know you're tired of repeating the same patterns because somewhere in your mind you know they're never going to get you "there." It's not because you're not working hard enough; it's because you're not slowing down, shutting out the noise, and listening to what your soul is trying to tell you. You're not looking at the data for what it is. You're missing all the messages. You're patchwork-solutioning your way through your health and wellness journey instead of feeling into what's right for you on the path to achieving your goals.

You *can* overcome the plight of perfection and still be a major achiever. It's not *easy*, but if you're willing to do the work, you really can get better at riding the wave of ups and downs, feeling good in your own skin, and achieving your goals in a realistic, healthy way. You can learn how to prioritize progress over perfection. Here's the difference between these mindsets:

WITH PERFECTION	WITH PROGRESS
You never get there.	You're already there.
You focus on fixing flaws.	You focus on improving strengths.
Results are about success or failure.	Results are about learning no matter what.
You focus on others.	You focus on yourself.
You are competitive.	You are collaborative.
You hate criticism.	You welcome feedback.
You have a scarcity mindset.	You have an abundance mindset.
You derive self-worth from success.	You derive self-worth from living in alignment with your values.
You are outcome driven.	You are process driven.
You manage time.	You manage energy.

It's time for you to set aside the judgment you carry with you at every stage of your journey in order to be able to celebrate strategy, effort, courage, and resilience. Only when you begin to do this will you be able to create a climate of progress rather than perfection.

REFLECT AND REMEMBER

Reflect

Do you feel ready to let go of some of the self-judgment that's been holding you to impossible standards? Are you committed to shifting your focus to more positive aspects of yourself and your journey going forward?

Remember

1. The amount of energy required to pursue perfection is exhausting and requires you to behave in a way that is totally contradictory to your biological and psychological programming.

2. Perfectionism *does not* have to reach torturous levels to negatively impact your life. Even milder forms of perfectionism can prevent you from achieving the momentum you're so desperately looking for.

3. If you can learn to celebrate strategy, effort, courage, and resilience, then you'll be well on your way to creating a climate of progress rather than a climate of perfection.

8
Mindset to Movement

ALRIGHT, FRIENDS, LET'S TAKE A deep breath and acknowledge the rather heavy shit you've been journeying through in this book so far.

You've discovered how your values drive you to spend your time in ways that support what's most important to you, and how becoming consciously aware of your values is crucial to breaking the on-again, off-again cycle. You've unpacked how your beliefs form the foundation of your expectations and determine your actions, and more importantly, how your limiting beliefs lead to self-sabotage when it comes to your health and wellness goals. You've also delved deep into the destructive nature of perfectionism, looking at how your fear and desire for control are holding you hostage in the unwavering pursuit of excellence.

It's been a lot.

I know.

I'm proud of you for staying the course.

These mindset shifts will set the stage for long-term, sustainable growth and transformation.

Now it's time to connect the "mind work" with the "body work" to practice manifesting your mindset shifts. This work is about the stuff that you can see, touch, and take control over as you break old patterns, refine a new way of living, and create a sense of momentum that will carry you through your journey.

And this part of the journey requires getting out of the passenger seat and into the driver's seat of your own life by influencing your thoughts and behaviors, taking control over your actions and their consequences, and having faith in your ability to handle what comes your way.

In other words, claiming your own agency.

Agency for how you want to feel.

Agency for the choices you make.

Agency for your commitment and follow-through, or lack thereof.

THERE IS NO MAGIC MINDSET SHIFT

Let's unpack the "I'll Start Again Tomorrow" narrative for a moment, because woven into it is the avoidance of taking agency *today*. It's this idea that "future you" will have more motivation, more commitment, and more resilience than "present you." It's this idea that "future you" will deal with the consequences and outcomes of the choices "present you" makes today. It's this idea that none of the things that caused you to fall off the wagon in the past will matter anymore, because "future you" will have somehow magically figured it all out.

You know the drill. You spend your weekend laying out an intense new regimen for yourself, and when Monday comes, you're on top of your shit. Workout at 6 a.m.? Done. Zero carbs all day? Easy. Then Tuesday comes and you start to feel a little wobbly. Halfway through the day, you *need* a snack, and those carrot sticks you prepped the night before are not cutting it. So you indulge in some dark chocolate and shrug it off. Or so you thought. Eventually, getting another bite of chocolate is all you can think of, and then suddenly you've eaten all of the snacks you can get your hands on, and you're at the start of a complete spiral. To ward off the feelings of intense guilt, you reassure yourself, saying that you'll start again tomorrow. But tomorrow comes and you just can't stop the spiral. It's the same the next day, and before you know it, it's Friday. And we all know, you can't possibly start fresh on a Friday. It's the end of the week, you're feeling drained and discouraged, you've completely lost touch with your goals. So you tell yourself something along the lines of:

"This coming Monday will be 'the Monday' that I'll finally be able to change my life."

All in.

So much hope.

So much fear.

So much pressure.

But here's the deal: your thoughts, feelings, and actions *today* set the stage for who you'll be tomorrow. There is no magic mindset shift that just happens when you decide "it's time." In order to *really* "do the work," you have to claim agency for how you *want* to feel, and then make choices that align with that future. We're all guilty of playing the blame game. Blaming our circumstances or our jobs or our relationships for our lack of follow-through. And no, I'm obviously not talking about those real moments of tragedy in life. Those moments happen. They're real. Because . . . well . . . life.

But here's what happens when you actually claim agency for how you want to feel—you show up to do the work that's actually required. Progressing from thought to action is the key to tapping into courage, commitment, and resilience. It's frankly the most critical piece in getting "unstuck." When I tapped into my sense of agency, I found everything became much clearer. Making decisions no longer felt as heavy because I understood, deep in my core, that I had to take action in order to experience a different reality. That I couldn't keep doing what I was doing the way I was doing it. That I had to choose differently in order to get back into the driver's seat of my life.

ACTION WITH INTENTION

Moving from your mind to your body is the first place to start manifesting your new mindset. This is where you practice detangling yourself from the #hashtag world, moving away from the Insta-reels that have you questioning if you're doing the right "top five things to maximize fat loss," and coming back to the real science and fundamentals of your body.

Cardio?

Carbs?

Core exercises?

We're stuck in the vortex. We have no clue anymore. We question our methods. We bounce from trend to trend, hoping something will get us closer to the body we so desperately want.

It's not about switching gears *away* from the mind work *to* the body work, but rather experiencing how the two mutually reinforcing approaches help you achieve better alignment. Mindset without movement is just an intention, and action without intention is aimless. We need both, and they need to be in sync. It's time to lay down a new foundation. To build a strong understanding of *what really matters* so that we can do things differently this time around. To unlearn everything that hasn't been serving us in order to get unstuck.

REFLECT AND REMEMBER

Reflect

Are you ready to get into the driver's seat of your own life? Are you ready to claim agency over your thoughts, behaviors, actions, and consequences in order to navigate the ups and downs of your journey?

Remember

1. You need to put your mindset shifts to work in order to break old patterns, refine a new way of living, and create a sense of *real* momentum.

2. Your thoughts, feelings, and actions *today* set the stage for who you'll be tomorrow. You have to claim agency for how you *want* to feel, and then make choices that align with that future.

3. You need to do the mind work to do the body work, and you need to do the body work to do the mind work. Mindset without movement is just an intention, and action without intention is aimless. You need both, and they need to be in sync so that you can achieve better alignment.

9

Your Body Is
a Smart Machine

THE #HASHTAG WORLD HAS DISTORTED our reality when it comes to nutrition. Everything is all about eating clean; drinking our greens; and having turmeric, chia, and flax on the daily. We doom-scroll social media, hunting for the best keto recipes when we don't actually *know* what keto is beyond the confusing "you have to eat fat to lose fat" statements floating around online. We hunt for the latest low-carb dessert inspiration, not knowing whether we actually *need* to be consuming fewer grams of carbs for our body type and metabolism. We (secretly) panic every time we see the latest TikTok trends replacing bread with lettuce and pasta with zucchini, because if we fail to follow suit, will that mean we don't want it badly enough?

It's a tough battle because there's so much misinformation out there. And so, we glue together mismatched pieces of the nutrition puzzle, hoping they'll stick with enough motivation and commitment. Without realizing it, perfectionism tightens its grip.

We dramatically cut calories (convincing ourselves that we're not hungry).

We cut out all carbs (believing deeply that bread is the enemy).

We get overly restrictive with our diet (swearing off anything that feels remotely indulgent).

It doesn't matter how we feel; we're in it to win it, and we're convinced that we'll "get back to normal eating" once we achieve our goals. But that day never comes. All we do is make ourselves feel like absolute shit until one day, we're fed up (but not actually fed at all), and decide to just *go for it*. We eat the burger and fries. We drink the Coke Zero. We eat the damn brownie, loving and hating every – single – bite.

And just like that, we find ourselves falling off the wagon. Just a little at first. Then we're in a full-fledged rebound.

WTF ARE CALORIES, ANYWAY?

Disclaimer: In this section, I'll be talking about calories and calorie intake in detail. If this is a trigger for you, feel free to skip forward.

Let's start by talking about the dreaded C word: "calories."

We know we don't like them. We know that we're scared of them.

But seriously, what *are* calories?

According to the Instagram memes, "calories are tiny creatures that live in our closets, sewing our clothes a little bit tighter every night."

According to the *Cambridge Dictionary*, the definition is:

Calorie: (n.) A unit of energy, often used as a measurement
of the amount of energy that food provides.[3]

Now, I'd like to offer some insight into the mysterious world of
calories so that you're no longer obsessing over a metric without even knowing *why* it matters to you or *how* it connects to
who you want to be.

Here's the deal: Eat too many calories and your body will
store the extra calories as fat. Eat fewer than you need and your
body will rely on its own energy stores to make up the difference, resulting in a net weight loss.

It's pretty simple, for the most part. And yet, there seems
to be a ton of confusion about whether, and to what extent,
calories determine if you gain or lose weight.

Let's move on to metabolism for a moment, another word
that leaves people feeling a little unsure of what's going on.
What is it and why does it matter?

Metabolism: (n.) The chemical and physical processes by
which a living thing uses food for energy and growth.[4]

We usually use the word "metabolism" interchangeably with
"metabolic rate," which is the number of calories you burn. The
higher your metabolic rate, the more calories you burn and the
easier it is to lose weight and keep it off.

THE FORMULA

To lose weight, you *must* create a calorie deficit. This means you need to burn more calories than you consume. You can do this by either moving more or eating less, neither of which sound all that fun, I know.

Now, bear with me for a moment as we get a bit "mathy." The most popular equation to determine a person's energy (calorie) needs accounts for sex, age, height, weight, and level of physical activity.

The equation for males is:
66.5 + 13.8 × (weight in kg) + 5 × (height in cm) - 6.8 × age

The equation for females is:
655.1 + 9.6 × (weight in kg) + 1.9 × (height in cm) - 4.7 × age

The results of these equations are then multiplied by an energy factor to determine estimated caloric needs. The energy factors are:

- 1.2 for sedentary people (desk job, no regular exercise)
- 1.3 for moderately active people (work out three times per week or work a non-desk job), and
- 1.4 for active people (work out five or six times per week or work a physically intense job)

If you didn't grow up in a household like mine, where testing your mental math skills was the norm (. . . thanks a lot, Dad), fear not: there are a ton of daily caloric calculators available online.

The average woman needs to consume 2,000 calories a day to maintain her weight. I know that sounds like a lot to most of you, because the #hashtag world has led us to think that we, as women, only need about 1,200 calories a day to be perfectly slim and trim.

But that's totally wrong.

You know who needs on average 1,200 calories a day? Five-year-old children, that's who. Take a moment. Let that sink in.

Now, to some of you, this may feel like a relief. But to some of you, your limiting beliefs may be acting up.

"Other women can eat 2,000 calories, but if I do, I'll definitely gain weight."

"If I start eating more, it'll just turn into a downward spiral of continuous eating."

"My metabolism is slower than other people's. The rules don't apply to me."

If you're finding the noise getting louder, this is an opportunity to practice the foundation we set earlier. Reflect back on your core values. Pull out your Mindset Manifesto. Broaden your focus beyond how you want to *look* to how you want to *feel.* Remind yourself of what's most important to you in order to begin rewriting your limiting beliefs about calories.

CALORIES ARE SNEAKY

I was thirty years old, and through a combination of post-partum anxiety, semi-healthy eating, and a gradual fitness regimen, I had lost my "baby weight." I was committed to "staying on track," but I was back at work and things were feeling really stressful on all fronts. Post-baby marriage. An actual baby. An evolving career that required a lot of mental and physical endurance. I wasn't spiraling out of control, but

I did start stress-snacking, taking in roughly 500 extra calories throughout the day. Nothing "unhealthy," though. God, no, I was still committed to my weight loss priorities. Just a skinny vanilla latte here, a Kashi granola bar there, and a pack of dry-roasted almonds to keep myself from falling apart. Week over week, my pants started to feel a smidge tighter around the waist. I started to (secretly) panic. "How can this be happening?!"

Well, as it turns out, I was gaining one pound of fat approximately every seven days thanks to my new snacking habits.

While 500 calories sounds like a lot, it's not necessarily a lot of food:

- One grande skinny vanilla latte equals 120 calories
- One Kashi granola bar equals 150 calories
- A single pouch of dry-roasted almonds equals 240 calories

That totals 510 calories.

Multiply this by seven days in a week, and you're looking at 3,500 calories, which is the equivalent of one pound of fat.

See how easy it is to eat an extra 500 calories per day without indulging in anything "unhealthy"? This is why you need to know your daily caloric requirement—you need to stop shooting in the dark, just hoping that you're within the correct range to achieve your goals.

This isn't about perfectionism, but metrics *do* matter. I want you to think of calorie counting not as a lifestyle but as a tool. And as with all tools, you need to understand the user manual in order to be responsible and safe. Take it from my decades of lived experience: without being mindful, it's easy to slip into subtle (but destructive) patterns of disordered eating. For some people, calorie counting *can* work for the long haul. For many of us, it's simply an important but brief phase to get clarity on how much energy our food provides us so that we can take aligned action toward achieving our goals and breaking through our limiting beliefs.

A SLIPPERY SLOPE

Let's say you need to eat 2,000 calories a day to maintain your weight. If you consistently eat more than that, just like I did, then you'll gain weight, "healthy eating" or not. But what happens when you consistently eat less than that?

At first, you'll lose weight because, as you know, a calorie deficit equals weight loss. But what happens when you continue to dip your calories lower and lower? Will you simply lose weight faster and faster? Nope. Instead, your body will catch on to the fact that it's starving and will adjust your metabolism accordingly. That's right. Your metabolism will *slow down* to conserve energy because you're not giving it enough fuel:

- Daily calorie requirement equals 2,000
- Daily consumption equals 1,500
- Daily deficit equals 500

Over one week, you lose one pound of fat. This continues for a while and you feel great about your progress. Then a few weeks later, your body catches on and your metabolism slows down. You don't panic, you simply dip your calories down even lower:

- New daily requirement equals 1,500
- Consumption equals 1,200
- Deficit equals 300

Over one week, you lose two-thirds of a pound of fat. The slower pace of fat loss doesn't feel ideal to you, but you're still optimistic that the pace will pick back up somehow. A few weeks later though, your body catches on again.

- New daily requirement equals 1,200
- Consumption equals 1,200
- Deficit equals 0

Over one week, you maintain your current weight, which is otherwise known as the dreaded "weight-loss plateau." You feel like shit about your lack of progress and start to panic but don't know what to do to fix the problem. How are you supposed to survive on less than 1,000 calories a day to keep your fat loss going? You try your best but inevitably throw in the towel out of frustration and fatigue.

And just like that, your weight-loss streak is over.

Sigh.

You can clearly see why you lose weight rapidly in the beginning and why it slows down as time goes on. Your body is smart: it catches on quickly and once it realizes that it's only going to be getting fewer calories than it needs, it slows itself down so that you don't . . . well, die.

So intelligent when you're trying to survive famine; so frustrating when you're trying to lose weight on purpose.

The real problem comes when you inevitably start eating *more* than 1,200 calories a day. Because it *will* happen. It always does. You know it as well as I do. Once you take your daily consumption back up to around 1,500 calories, you're now dealing with a daily 300-calorie surplus. This means suddenly you're gaining weight from eating 1,500 calories, whereas before you would have been losing weight while eating 1,500 calories. I know this sounds weirdly confusing, but remember, you needed 2,000 calories previously. Although 1,500 calories would have been a 500-calorie deficit then, you slowed your metabolism down to only need 1,200 calories.

The net result? You, my friend, are gaining weight eating even less than you were before you started your diet.

Holy shit.

F*CK OFF, FAD DIETS

There are ways to keep your metabolism revved up so that it doesn't slow down as quickly when you reduce your caloric intake. These strategies include staying hydrated, consuming more protein with your meals, increasing your muscle mass, getting sufficient sleep, and cycling your calories. These strategies *don't* include any of the fad diets and quick-fix solutions you're bombarded with in the #hashtag world.

Many of the standard starvation diets, detox teas, and juice cleanses that you see promoted online have you eating significantly less than you should, which leads to a whole slew of issues:

- Much of the weight you initially lose is water, which comes back freakishly quickly.

- You begin to lose muscle mass, and the less you eat, the more you lose.

- Your metabolism slows down and your bone health decreases.

- You experience a negative hormonal response, including: a decrease in thyroid hormone, which plays a key role in metabolism and declines with prolonged dieting; an increase in cortisol, a stress hormone that can cause many health issues and plays a role in fat gain when levels are constantly elevated; a decrease in leptin, which is an important hunger hormone that is supposed to tell your brain that you're full and to stop eating; an increase in ghrelin, a hormone produced in the digestive tract and that signals your brain that you're hungry.

You begin to feel like shit. Your energy levels drop. You battle intense food cravings. You become mentally cloudy and, frankly, all around hangry.

These adaptations are the exact opposite of what you need for successful, long-term weight loss, and this is if you're even *able* to stick with such a large deficit for long enough. Most people can't, and frankly, that's a good thing because starving yourself is the worst. I did it for years. It takes a major toll. You know all those diets like keto and intermittent fasting that you see promoted across your feed? Honestly, they're all just deliberate ways to create a deep calorie deficit. That's it.

For example, the reason calorie counting isn't usually necessary on a ketogenic diet is that when you keep your carbohydrate and sugar intake low, your protein intake moderately high, and your fat intake super-high, you experience a natural decrease in appetite. Fat and protein keep you full longer so that you don't want to eat as much as frequently. Thus, your daily caloric intake decreases pretty much on its own.

The same goes for intermittent fasting, which is another hot topic these days. This is one strategy that seems to "take the thinking out of eating" because you can eat whatever you want within an eight-hour window as long as you're fasting for the other sixteen. Why does this work? Well, it's hard for people to eat as much as they typically do in twelve hours when they have only eight "sanctioned hours" available to them. Yes, there is a whole bunch of supporting evidence for the beneficial hormonal shifts that come along with intermittent fasting, but the primary factor remains the same: your daily caloric intake needs to decrease for a diet to be an effective method of weight loss.[5]

If your goal is weight loss, then you need to be aware of calories even when fasting or following a ketogenic diet. If you *do* end up frequently eating more calories than your body needs, even if those calories don't come from carbs, then those calories *will* get stored as body fat. There's just no way around this phenomenon.

So, if you're focused on fat loss, my suggestion is to reduce your caloric intake by 15 to 20 percent to see weekly results while preserving your metabolic health, energy balance, mood, and commitment. Of course, 15 to 20 percent is a general guideline. The best way to truly individualize your deficit is to:

1. Identify how quickly you can lose weight while maintaining muscle.

2. Identify how large a deficit you can realistically sustain—physically, mentally, and emotionally.

3. Use steps one and two to give you an appropriate caloric deficit.

The bottom line is this: you have to know your daily caloric requirement and manage your intake accordingly.

LIMITING BELIEF
I have to try all the trending diets until
I find one that works for me.

NEW BELIEF
I ignore the trends and focus on simple science.

FUN AND FLEXIBILITY

A great way to manage your caloric intake, while also creating a better foundation for a sustainable mindset, is to implement caloric cycling.

> Calorie cycling: (n.) A dieting style that allows you to cycle between lower-calorie and higher-calorie periods.[6]

Because total fat loss doesn't necessarily depend on how many calories you eat on a specific day but rather on creating a total calorie deficit over time, it's possible to alternate days of calorie deficits and calorie surpluses and still lose body fat. What's even better, by cycling your calories, you may be less likely to lose muscle mass, slow down your metabolism, and fall into a fat-loss plateau. This practice can be especially effective if you match your high-calorie days to the days when you're strength training, because your body will use the extra fuel for your workouts and recovery. The best part, though? You'll have some wiggle room in your diet so that you can *enjoy* the food you love without all the negative narrative that often comes along with it.

I was twenty-two years old and had just moved back home after finishing university. My brother was getting married at the end of the summer and I *really* wanted to lose weight so that I could feel more "confident" in a sari. At the time, I needed to eat 2,000 calories a day, or 14,000 calories per week. In order to lose a pound of fat a week, I needed to create a deficit of 3,500 calories (reminder: one pound of fat equals 3,500 calories). I exercised more, I ate less, and I managed to come in each day at 1,500 calories per day.

- Monday: 1,500
- Tuesday: 1,500
- Wednesday: 1,500
- Thursday: 1,500
- Friday: 1,500
- Saturday: 1,500
- Sunday: 1,500
- Total: 10,500

Needs: 14,000
Consumed: 10,500
Deficit = 3,500 = one pound fat

As you can see, my total calories for the week were 10,500, which landed me perfectly in my sweet spot to lose one pound per week.

But then I began my career as an account executive in the corporate world. I was faced with several client dinners each week, and while I was committed to keeping my regimen on track and making healthy choices as much as I could, I began to struggle. The occasional cocktail or two here, a delicious piece of warm bread or dessert there. Suddenly, I was veering away from my goals and my perfect track record started to feel tarnished. I couldn't figure out a way to keep my progress going. I started to waver—just slightly at first, but then it became an all-out free fall.

If only I had known about calorie cycling—a concept I came to learn about and love later in life.

Instead of falling off the wagon, I could have simply decided to cycle my calories throughout the week in order to better accommodate my client dinners, while *still* staying on track to lose one pound a week.

My road map could have looked like some version of this:

- Monday: 1,500
- Tuesday: 1,850
- Wednesday: 1,150
- Thursday: 1,600
- Friday: 1,400
- Saturday: 1,900
- Sunday: 1,100
- Total: 10,500

I would still have ended the week with a 3,500-calorie deficit, but I'd have achieved it by cycling my calories up and down versus keeping them steady day over day.

Can you see how this method allows for a lot more variation and lets you better manage your social calendar? You can accommodate corporate dinners, celebrations, and the simple need to "eat more today" without feeling like you're damaging your progress. It's been a game-changer for me, helping pacify my perfectionist tendencies and allowing me to "go with the flow" a little more. Oh, we're going out for a last-minute dinner? No problem. I'll just shift how I'm cycling my calories for the week without all the negative narrative and angst, and just like that, I'm still in control of my journey. And when I indulge,

I enjoy it to the fullest: no negative mental chatter, no guilt, no overthinking, and no buyer's remorse. I decide what I want to eat and then I simply enjoy it.

Why? Because I know that less nutrient-dense foods are a part of my plan. I know that I'm not getting carried away or falling off track. I know that one cupcake no longer has the power to derail me.

PERFECT DOESN'T EXIST

The purpose of calorie cycling is to stave off the noticeable negative effects of dieting, like decreased energy, weaker gym performance, and the dreaded fat-loss plateau. However, there are no definitive rules for calorie cycling.

This is about *your* mindset.

It all comes down to what *you* value.

Your metrics of success.

If you're someone who values structure and routine, you may want to consistently stick with a lower-calorie period for two to four weeks, then layer in five to seven days of higher-calorie eating. This structure is an excellent way to keep your metabolism revved up while ensuring that you don't feel like you're tipping on the brink of insanity. On the other hand, if you're someone who values a more intuitive mind-body connection, you may choose to simply listen to your body to understand when to give yourself a few days of refuel before your next "structured block." This method is a great way to practice flow and flexibility.

Here are a few calorie-cycling protocols to consider:

- **Weekend cycle.** Five days on a low-calorie diet followed by two days of higher-calorie eating.

- **Mini cycle.** Eleven days on a low-calorie diet followed by three days of higher-calorie eating.

- **Three on, one off.** Three weeks on a low-calorie diet followed by five to seven days of higher-calorie eating.

- **Monthly cycle.** Four to five weeks on a low-calorie diet followed by a longer ten-to-fourteen-day higher-calorie refeed.

LIMITING BELIEF
I can't lose weight because I don't have the
discipline to eat healthy 100 percent of the time.

NEW BELIEF
I follow a "healthy eating protocol" that is realistic
and allows me to enjoy the foods I love in moderation.

80/20 FOR THE WIN!

Calorie cycling is a great strategy for fat loss, but what if it feels too complicated, or you're not interested in getting so specific? Then I would suggest that you adopt the 80/20 rule: a minimum of 80 percent of your week follows your "healthy eating protocol" and a maximum of 20 percent of your week is made up of fun, flexible eating. While 20 percent may not sound like a lot, it adds up to about four meals per week where you can take your foot off the gas pedal. Yes, it's great to be passionate about your goals, but if your path to achieving them is so rigid that it doesn't allow for some fun, then maybe your goals are actually just restrictions in your life.

Now, fun should feel more like a splurge than a binge, in my opinion. I don't use my flexible meals as an opportunity to eat the equivalent of 15,000 calories in one sitting. I allow myself a plate of pasta and some dessert, or a burger and a cookie. I don't eat three burgers paired with a milkshake, chocolate cake, and wine. So, yes, treat yourself and enjoy it, but the word is still "moderation."

BREAK IT DOWN

I know, you're busy. You have work, commitments, relation-ships, and children. Coming home from a hard day of work and then masterfully creating a delicious, healthy meal can be a reality for some, but for many it's not. If you're anything like me, you just don't have the time and energy during the week to care. You need something quick and easy, something that may not win you a place on *Master Chef* but will at least taste better than cardboard. And sometimes you're so busy it's just easier to pick something up or order in.

But each meal matters. Remember, we're talking about making good choices at least 80 percent of the time. That means you're eating well about six days of the week. In some ways, weekdays are the easiest time to keep things on point because we want to eat and drink and have all the fun on the weekends. However, this puts the onus on you to be organized about your weekdays.

Pick a day to map out your week, buy the groceries you need for your meals, and prep whatever you can so that your week is that much easier. Your meal prep doesn't have to look Pinterest-pretty for the #hashtag world; it just has to get done. Some people do the bulk of their cooking on Sunday and then freeze their food for the week so that all they have to do is take their dinner out of the freezer when they get home. Some people don't like leftovers or defrosting food, so they just have their recipes ready to go. It doesn't matter which approach you take as long as you're organized and structured about it, so you don't accidentally end up eating lasagna three days in a row.

REFLECT AND REMEMBER

Reflect

What is your primary focus, nutrition or calories? Are you the type of person who needs to create firm rules around "eating healthy" to feel like you're on track? Or are you more comfortable with an approach that focuses solely on calories?

Remember

1. Calories provide your body with energy. If you eat more than you need, you'll gain weight. If you consume less than you need, you'll lose weight (for a while).

2. Calculating your caloric requirement doesn't have to be a pain in the ass. Google "daily caloric requirement" and input your data into one of the many calculators you'll find. It'll take you a total of two minutes, I promise!

3. You don't have to eat kale to keep your calories in check, although eating clean, wholesome foods can certainly make managing your caloric intake easier.

10
Feeding the Machine

NOW ON TO *WHAT* YOU should eat. If you're feeling lost, you're not alone. It seems like the facts are changing minute to minute these days. It also seems like every other person who pops up on your feed has an opinion about what you should or shouldn't be eating.

Fat is bad.
No wait, now fat is good. It's carbs that are bad.
No wait, now carbs are good, it's actually wheat that is bad.
Wait, but isn't whole wheat supposed to be good for you? Isn't dairy the culprit we're after?
Or sugar? Yes, sugar is definitely bad for you.
But what about fruit? Aren't you supposed to eat, like, several servings a day?

Understanding the fundamentals of nutrition is vital to practicing and refining your new mindset as well as ensuring your body is getting exactly what it needs. You need to be clear on the facts to feel empowered and in charge of your daily actions.

Contrary to popular opinion, you *can* achieve your goals without eating healthy food. You can eat McDonald's for all your meals and make it happen. It's pretty hard, but it *can* be done if you carefully manage how many calories you're taking in each day. Except this is obviously a terrible idea, so please don't. Really, don't.

Alternatively, you can choose to eat clean to keep your calories in check.

Here's the reality: It's harder to gain fat on lean chicken, brown rice, steel-cut oats, and egg whites because they contain fewer calories than, let's say, the same volume of pizza. Two slices of pepperoni pizza will run you around 900 calories, give or take. That's the equivalent of two heaping cups of brown rice and a pound of chicken. Same number of calories but a *huge* difference in volume. Two slices of pizza are pretty easy to eat. Let's be honest, I can easily eat three or four. But a mountain of rice and a pound of chicken? Not so much.

Your diet will literally make or break your progress. But what does "diet" really mean?

Does it mean salad (without salad dressing) and chicken (without seasoning) three times a day? Does it mean cutting your calories from 2,000 to 1,000?

Does it mean overdosing on protein bars until you can't stand the taste of faux chocolate any longer?

When determining what to include in your diet, you need to decide whether nutrition or overall calorie count matters most to you. There's *seriously* no right or wrong answer here, but clarifying your evaluation criteria will help you make the right food choices to support your goals.

I get that it's confusing. I spent years of my life spinning myself in circles.

YO-YO DIETING

It all started in my teens. On day one of high school, I tried this thing called a "panzerotti," and let's just say it was the beginning of the end. I got a taste of deep-fried dough, tomato sauce, pepperoni, and cheese . . . oh, so much cheese . . . and I was forever changed. It was the start of my first real weight rebound—the first time I ever really ate my way to a bigger size. I gained fifteen pounds over the course of a few months, and I loved/hated every minute of it.

Fast-forward to university, where I put the traditional "frosh fifteen" to shame by gaining an impressive thirty-five pounds in my first year alone. Every day, three times a day, I was essentially at an all-you-can-eat buffet filled with pizza and burgers and quesadillas. In the beginning, I just wanted to try a little bit of everything because "I deserved it." I had finally made it to university, and it was my time to have fun. That, in and of itself, was enough to keep my weight gain going. Then, after my enthusiasm for salty food finally waned, I moved over to the sugary cereal quadrant of the cafeteria, where I discovered the delicious likes of Lucky Charms, Corn Pops, and Cinnamon Toast Crunch. Coupled with the dessert buffet that practically threw itself at me . . . Well, let's just say my waistline didn't stand a chance.

Yes, I was eating for the fun of it because I liked food, and it was delicious, and I was excited by my newfound freedom. But there was also some other very real shit at play. I went to university thinking that I would finally be in my sweet spot, that all the "struggling to be good enough" stuff would be behind me and that I'd finally hit my stride. Turns out, I had grossly overestimated my intellect and grossly underestimated the program I was in. Before I knew it, I was trapped in panic-survival mode. I was chronically anxious about getting mediocre grades. I was desperately hungry for success (and cake). I was totally out of touch with my personal evaluation criteria, coping the only way I knew how in order to get to the "end destination." It wasn't about the journey at all.

And so, I stress-ate my face off for an entire year. I studied till the wee hours of the morning and then ate a slice of pizza at 3 a.m. I woke up feeling anxious about school, so I ate a muffin, or two. I stress-ate to pacify the anxious voices in my head, and all I had to do was wear baggy sweatpants and an oversized hoodie to silence the other voice in my head that was saying, "Hey, you're getting, like, way bigger. *Ew.*" Despite my best efforts, though, in my first year of university, I was only able to pull off high seventies, low eighties, and a solid failing grade in Accounting 101. You can imagine what that did to my parents, and what it did to the perfectionist in me. I was devastated that I, "Mediocre Sonia," had gone to university and failed a course. I had done the unthinkable.

Luckily, the university staff could see that I was dealing with some rather extenuating circumstances ("self-inflicted chronic anxiety") and didn't kick me out of the program. I was put on probation, I had to repeat Accounting 101, and I was given a second chance to show my worth. I went home during the summer after my first year of university scared shitless of how disappointed my parents were but also more determined than ever to succeed. Sure, I had gone and messed up my first year of university. Sure, I couldn't recognize myself in the mirror. But I wasn't going to let that stop me. I was determined to take back control. I wanted to *feel* like I was in charge of my life. I needed to *know* that I could do it. And the first action item on my "quest to succeed" list? Losing all the weight I had gained. It was the one area of my life where I felt like I could really take responsibility for everything that had happened throughout the year.

The weight loss happened surprisingly fast. I think it took me about two months of pretty religious diet and exercise. Then I went back to my old plan of becoming "fit" and not just "skinny," and so I started dabbling in weights in addition to doing regular bouts of intense cardio. For the first time in my life, I started to see the benefits of strength training. Not only was I getting skinnier faster by lifting weights, but my body composition was changing as well. I could see a teeny bit of definition head to toe. I was by no means "fit" like I wanted to be, but thanks to a little bit of strength training, I spent the summer feeling pretty strong, and kind of beautiful. But here's the truth of the matter: I was achieving physical results without healing my mindset. The "results" were fleeting. One minute I was so on track, I couldn't even understand how I'd existed any other way, and the next minute I was quietly swearing to myself that I'd "start again tomorrow." I was stuck in the vortex because I hadn't actually overcome my limiting beliefs, perfectionist tendencies, and self-sabotaging behavior. I failed again and again and again.

The rest of my university career was rather predictable. I learned how to study, I worked smarter instead of harder, I got eighties and nineties in my classes and landed myself on the dean's list. As for my weight? From second to fourth year, I continued the same old cycle. I'd gain about five to ten pounds during stressful times of the year, like during midterms, large case study projects, and finals. Then I'd wear myself out for a month, hitting the gym and dieting super-hard, vowing that I would be different once the excess weight came off. I was your classic yo-yo girl, bouncing back and forth by ten pounds in either direction. It was just enough of a swing to have me going from "obviously thin" to "kind of chunky depending on the outfit."

Inevitably, I'd always fall off the wagon and eat myself back to my original size.

In these phases, I'd eat everything. Like, really: All. The. Things. Every single thing that I had deprived myself of. I wouldn't just indulge in a little treat here or there. No, I would eat everything, all the time, because I knew that this phase would be temporary. Soon I'd be back in "regimen mode," and then I wouldn't be allowed to eat anything again. It was either now or never. Again and again, I'd start my fitness regimen, I'd love it, I'd thrive off it, I'd overdo it, I'd fall off, I'd eat myself sick, I'd gain ten pounds, and . . . *repeat.* The battle (secretly) consumed my soul.

For years, I was in a loop of yo-yo dieting, of following the (often contradictory) advice from random people on my feed, of trying new (and honestly exhausting) diets. I was left feeling drained, foggy, and physically and mentally exhausted. It was only when I muted the outside noise and went back to the basic facts was I able to break my cycle. And a key part of the process was fueling my body with what it needed—clean, nourishing foods.

You probably have a general sense of what I mean when I say, "eat clean." But let me clarify exactly what it entails since buzzword concepts like "eating clean" are often made out to be infinitely more complicated than they really are.

FRUIT AND VEGETABLES

If it falls from a tree or comes from the ground, then it's safe to say it's a good, clean choice. I know you get the gist of why there's so much hype around veggies, so I won't waste your time reinforcing what you already know: veggies are awesome. They're full of good things, and you should eat as many as you can as often as you can.

Let's talk about fruit for a minute, since popular "diet news" floating around online has led people to think that eating fruit will make you fat. In a nutshell? False. Both fruits and vegetables are a good source of vitamins and minerals, as well as dietary fiber, which can help maintain a healthy gut, prevent digestive problems, and keep you regular. They're also low in fat and calories, which can help you maintain a healthy weight.

Yes, there's a lot of evidence about how harmful added sugar can be to the body. But this doesn't apply to whole fruits. Fructose, the sugar found in fruit, is harmful only in excessive amounts, which is difficult to get from consuming whole fruit because, let's face it, unlike a bag of gummies, fruit is seriously hard to overeat.[7] In general, fruit is just a minor source of fructose in a diet compared with added sugars, so consider yourself safe. As far as I know, nobody has ever gained weight by eating too many apples.

IS JUICE A FRUIT?

What about juicing or smoothies, you ask? Cold-pressed juices and smoothies are all the rage these days, but unfortunately, eating fruit and drinking juice aren't the same thing. The key difference is that juices lack fiber. Juicing releases the sugars in fruit and removes the insoluble fiber; similarly, blending fruit releases the sugars and tears apart the insoluble fiber. Why is this a problem? Well, a small amount of fructose (like that found in an apple for example) does us no harm because we consume it along with the fiber present in the fruit as a whole. This fiber slows down the absorption of the fructose and makes us feel full. Fruit juices, on the other hand, don't have any fiber left in them at all, so we absorb the sugar immediately.

Some experts say that drinking fructose in liquid form stops the liver from doing its job properly, which can cause a whole range of health problems, including obesity, type 2 diabetes, and increased fat production.[8]

Fructose also fools our brains into thinking that we're still hungry, even when we're not. It's addictive, makes us crave more, and can cause us to overeat.

If you're going to incorporate juice into your diet, here are some things you can do to stave off the negative effects:

- Make your own so that you can control what goes into it.
- Limit your intake to a couple of glasses a week as a simple nutritional top up.
- Blend instead of juice—you'll retain more fiber this way.
- Focus on vegetables and use only a handful of fruit.

- Consider adding the juice of half a lemon to cut the taste of the vegetables without adding more sugar.
- Add fat, like avocado or flaxseed, to slow the absorption of sugars.

PROTEIN

If you're not a vegetarian, then lean meats are a fantastic source of protein. Eating more protein has been shown to reduce muscle loss and the subsequent drop in metabolism often associated with dieting and losing fat. Eating any food increases your metabolism for a few hours because of the extra calories required to digest, absorb, and process the nutrients from your meal. This is known as the thermic effect of food. Protein, however, causes the largest increase in your metabolic rate: 15 to 30 percent, compared with 5 to 10 percent for carbs and 0 to 3 percent for fats.[9]

One small note, however, because "more" is not always better: while protein is fantastic, you want to make sure you're balancing your protein intake with enough fiber, otherwise you'll be left feeling pretty constipated.

No need to panic if you're a vegetarian; there are many great ways for you to take advantage of protein's benefits, too. Legumes such as beans and peas, non-GMO tofu, seitan, pea protein, TVP (textured vegetable protein), greens such as broccoli and brussels sprouts, rice, and nuts are all great vegetarian options.

HEALTHY FATS

This one is my favorite. I spent 90 percent of my life being fat-phobic, eating anything and everything fat-free in sight, and it got me nowhere. Not only did I fail to achieve long-lasting results, but also most of the faux-health food I consumed until the age of twenty-five tasted pretty shitty. Instead of adopting a low-fat diet like I did, focus on eating beneficial "good" fats and avoiding harmful "bad" fats:[10]

- **"Good" unsaturated fats.** Monounsaturated and polyunsaturated fats can lower disease risk. Foods high in good fats include avocados, nuts, seeds, and fish.

- **"Bad" fats.** Trans fats can increase disease risk, even when eaten in small quantities. Trans fats are primarily found in processed foods made from partially hydrogenated oil such as fried fast foods, baked goods, and candy bars.

- **Saturated fats.** While not as harmful as trans fats, saturated fats can also negatively impact health and are best consumed in moderation. Foods containing large amounts of saturated fat include red meat, butter, cheese, and ice cream.

Good fats help you stay full longer, keep your hormones in balance, and control your blood sugar. You also need fat to absorb certain nutrients, such as fat-soluble vitamins (vitamins A, D, E, and K) and antioxidants (like lycopene and beta-carotene). In addition, omega-3 fats, a type of unsaturated fat, are important for optimum nerve, brain, and heart function.

GRAINS

Contrary to what the #hashtag world has you believing, carbs are not the enemy if you pick the right ones. Whole grains good for weight loss include brown rice, whole oats, unhulled barley, and quinoa; these grains have not gone through the grinding or processing of their kernels into flour. When whole grain kernels are ground into flour, they're a danger to our waistlines. Pick good carbs that take longer to digest, and your body will thank you.

Let's compare brown rice to white rice: brown rice is essentially what rice is supposed to look like when it's not refined and stripped of its natural goodness. Brown rice has amazing things like fiber, protein, thiamine, calcium, magnesium, and potassium. White rice, on the other hand, pretty much has nothing.[11] Yes, the calorie content is the same, but with white rice, your body won't really be able to use the food for anything productive.

LIMITING BELIEF
Eating carbs will make me fat.

NEW BELIEF
Carbs fuel my body with energy and provide me with much-needed nutrients, so long as I pick the right ones!

NO JUDGMENT

A gentle recommendation? Eat fewer packaged goods. Just because they claim to be healthy doesn't mean they are. Marketing really messes shit up. You should also avoid foods labeled "fat-free," because they are laden with extra sugar and chemicals. If it sounds too good to be true, it probably is.

The bottom line is this: Get clear on your personal evaluation criteria. What do you *really* care about? Nutrition? Calories? Moderation? There is no right answer. Regardless of what you value, total compliance isn't necessary, and if eating clean isn't realistic for you, then it isn't the way to go. Period. I don't care what any diet out there says. The point isn't to shame yourself for eating foods that aren't on some generic "sanctioned list" but rather for you to make clear, confident nutrition choices based on your body's needs and the things that matter most to you. It isn't about one single food but rather about your diet as a whole, because any food in excess is *not* the way to go. Yes, that even includes kale. It's your diet, collectively and consistently, across time that will dictate your results. Nutrition isn't a religion, and food trends will come and go no matter what the random influencers say. Ultimately, your approach to food is something that should be very personal to you. No judgment.

I'LL JUST HAVE WATER, THANKS

I have a love-hate relationship with this principle. On the one hand, I know just how important and valuable water is to the body and so I'm like, "Yes, drink more!" On the other hand, I personally just *don't like* drinking water for a few, very legitimate reasons: I don't like the taste of it. I don't like having to pee all the time. I really like the taste of Coke Zero.

But water is *so* important when you're on any kind of "get fit" journey. We all know that roughly 70 percent of the body is made up of water. But you may not know that:

- Bone consists of 22 percent water.
- Muscle consists of 75 percent water.
- Blood consists of 83 percent water.
- The brain consists of 85 percent water.[12]

It's no wonder that water plays such a huge part in our health and well-being. We're literally made up of it. Water is crucial for proper body function, which is why I personally drink at least two liters a day. Here are some other ways in which hydration is key for optimal health.

Water is essential for proper digestion and nutrient absorption.[13] If you take the time and energy to refine your diet, then you also must emphasize your water intake to maximize your body's ability to transport and absorb nutrients. What's the point of eating nutrient-dense foods if your body can't reap the benefits?

Our metabolisms also require an adequate supply of water in order to function efficiently. Dehydration slows down the metabolism and therefore inhibits the calorie/fat-burning process. Lifting weights until you're blue in the face won't do you any good if you're not drinking enough water.

The body's metabolic process creates toxins, and water plays a critical role in flushing them out of your system. Thinking about doing a "detox" or a "cleanse"? Why don't you first try drinking enough water and let your liver and kidneys do what they're meant to do?

Fiber is a vital part of a healthy diet, but we often forget that fiber requires adequate fluid to pass through your system. I know I'm not alone when I say that I am a happier and friendlier human being when I can poop easily and regularly.

Most people aren't all that good at reading their body's signals. In fact, most people (including myself) often confuse thirst with hunger. What does this mean? It means that we're in danger of taking in extra calories for no reason! It may sound silly, but I drink a glass of water every time I start to feel unexpected hunger pangs. Nine times out of ten, I'm just thirsty.

LIMITING BELIEF
I'll never be skinny because I'm not hardcore enough to do a week-long juice cleanse. That takes real commitment, which I clearly don't have.

NEW BELIEF
My body needs basic support to detoxify itself. By drinking water, I'm already on track.

There you have it: five straightforward reasons to start drinking more water immediately. If you're feeling sluggish despite getting good sleep, if you're not seeing the fat loss you'd expect despite paying close attention to your diet, or if you're simply finding that your mouth is dry more often than not, toss out your Coke Zero and drink some water. Commit to drinking an extra five hundred milliliters a week and take it from there. Yes, the peeing will drive you nuts for a while... but stay strong; it'll pass (pun intended).

REFLECT AND REMEMBER

Reflect

Does this feel like the right time to prioritize nutrition in your life? Why or why not? Is there any resistance that comes up when you think about fueling your body with clean foods?

Remember

1. Fruit, fat, and carbs aren't the enemy. You just have to pick the right ones to reap the benefits. Good fat is particularly important, so don't fall for all the fat-free crap out there!

2. Protein is key if you want to prevent muscle loss and keep your metabolic rate strong.

3. Water will never taste like Coke Zero, but it's crucial you drink it anyway. It's fundamental to your health and wellness journey.

11

Ditch Your Stupid Scale

I CAN'T TELL YOU HOW many people have shared this frustration with me: every day, they start their morning by stepping onto the scale, and every day, their scale says they're not getting any smaller.

I also can't tell you how frustrated I get hearing shit like this, because I know for a fact that the scale is a stupid, stupid, stupid machine.

Why?

THE SCALE IS STUPID: REASON ONE

How many of you have set a weight goal only to hit that specific number and still not be satisfied with what you look like? I've been there. Many times. I naturally have flat glutes and boxy shoulders; that's just how I'm built. No number on the scale will ever guarantee that those features will change. Here's the deal: the scale doesn't account for the unique shape of your body, which is determined by genetics. Just because you weigh a certain amount doesn't mean your proportions are going to reflect your desired look. You may be top-heavy, you may be bottom-heavy, or you may not lose weight from the areas you are most concerned about. So, the number on the scale is irrelevant, and instead you need to get clear on your values. Do you actually want to hit a certain weight? Is the number really what's most important to you?

Or have you, in fact, been chasing something else entirely this whole time?

THE SCALE IS STUPID: REASON TWO

Many of my clients fear the number on the scale because it doesn't align with what the #hashtag world has trained them to believe their magic number should be. They want so badly to be 120 pounds because diet culture has told them that a slim and trim woman must weigh no more than that. However, for their height and body frame, that weight just may not be realistic.

Have you ever found yourself fixating on some "magic number"? And when you see the number on your scale going up, do you panic? Here's the deal: you think you're getting fatter or bulkier when in reality, the scale is telling you nothing relevant about your body composition. What's even worse is that as you lean down and pack on muscle, the number on the scale often starts to go up. Why? Because muscle weighs more than fat by volume. Yes, you heard me, the scale can *go up* even when you're *leaning down*. I'm sure you see the problem here.

If you're still depending on the scale to be your primary measure of progress, then it's time for a reframe. Dig deep and ask yourself:

How am I deriving my self-worth from the scale?

Why do the numbers mean so much to me?

How can I practice pivoting my perspective?

THE SCALE IS STUPID: REASON THREE

I know so many people who weigh themselves a few times a week (most do it daily) and freak out when the scale goes up by a couple of pounds. They become emotional, sad, and disheartened. Ultimately, they feel like quitting. But here's the thing—there are so many reasons for the number on the scale to fluctuate:

- Higher sodium intake in a snack or meal
- A "treat" meal
- Soreness post-workout
- Bowel movements

All these factors can and do increase water retention, which ultimately makes the scale go up. But have you gained any real weight? Have you gained any fat? Are you any larger? No. No. No.

When you rely on the scale to guide your self-perception, you fuel a cycle of self-sabotage. When you step on the scale and see that the number is higher, you panic and let your limiting beliefs take over. Don't be a slave to the scale—it's only one very narrow piece of information, and it's likely holding you back.

LIMITING BELIEF
*I'm a failure because I see that the number
on the scale has gone up.*

NEW BELIEF
*I know that the scale can play all sorts of mind-games
with me. I rely on other (reliable) methods to track my progress
and evaluate whether I need to make any changes.*

There are so many more accurate ways to gauge your progress than the scale. The question is, what *really* matters to you?

If you're tracking size, you might consider taking measurements with a measuring tape for maximum accuracy. If this doesn't sound appealing to you, I get it. I don't measure myself either, because doing so really amplifies my perfectionist tendencies. We all have that pair of jeans we use as our "anchor" for what we want to look like. My suggestion? Use those jeans as your benchmark so that you don't have to rely on how you "think" you're doing.

If you're monitoring aesthetics, track your progress with pictures. I still suffer from body dysmorphia—yes, even to this day—so I always look in the mirror and see someone bigger looking back at me. Pictures make reality clearer so that my limiting beliefs and perfectionist tendencies can't overtake my sanity.

If you're more interested in performance, set new benchmarks for yourself and challenge yourself at regular intervals. Track your progress and celebrate your wins. This is a great way to shift your focus away from the false "numbers game" the scale makes us play.

At the end of the day, it doesn't matter what you decide to focus on. Everyone is different and so we'll all set different goals for ourselves. The key is that these are *your* goals, not the goals that you've been influenced into believing are import-ant. So, get rid of the scale. It's not serving you the way your authentic values and evaluation criteria can (and will!).

REFLECT AND REMEMBER

Reflect

Do you feel ready to detach from your scale? If not, what's hold-ing you back? What feels realistic for you—can you "scale back" on your use of the scale to once a week to begin with? Then evolve from there?

Remember

1. Get rid of your scale.

2. See number one.

3. See number one.

12

The Heavy Lift, Literally

JUST AS WE'VE SEEN WITH the nutrition side of the equation, the #hashtag world has also convoluted our perspective on fitness. We bounce from interval training, to fasted cardio, to heavy lifting, to CrossFit, in the hopes that we'll crack the code on "rapid fat loss." We work out seven days a week to prove to ourselves that "we really want it." We do crunches till we're blue in the face to pacify our angst around belly fat. We chase fitness in the hopes that we'll one day look like the beautiful fitness influencers online, so that we, too, will one day be . . . happy.

When we think of nutrition, we often think about cutting things out of our diet. Forbidden foods. Things to avoid at all costs. On the other hand, when we think of fitness, we think of exhausting effort. Pushing ourselves. Doing as much as possible as frequently as possible.

But what would happen if we were to slow down for a moment and reconnect with ourselves?

What would happen if we stopped chasing fitness and instead viewed movement as yet another aspect of *living* our mindset? What would happen if we approached our exercise philosophy as an extension of who we *really* are?

Fitness isn't about constraints and limitations. It's about potential—learning to work with your body, not against it, in order to achieve better inner-outer alignment. It's about discovering how movement can *feel good* and then showing up to do it in whatever way feels most authentic to you. It's about connecting with your strength and endurance and flexibility and power because each of these elements makes up *who you are.*

It's time to get clear on the facts so that you can put your mindset into action.

GET OFF THE TREADMILL

Have you ever thought to yourself, "Let me shed the fat first by doing cardio, and then I'll build the muscle after with weights"?

Mmhmm. I've been there.

There's no polite way to say this, so I'm just going to say it—you're doing it *totally* wrong.

The reality is that muscle directly affects your metabolism, and your metabolism directly affects how rapidly you can lose weight. The more muscle you have, the faster your metabolism will be, which means you'll lose weight much faster than someone with a slower metabolism. There's a strong misconception that "cardio is for fat loss," when cardio is, in fact, less effective than resistance training.

Relax, I'm not saying don't do any cardio. You're right, there are lots of great benefits to doing cardio:

- It makes your heart strong so that the muscle doesn't have to work as hard to pump blood.
- It increases your lung capacity.
- It helps reduce your risk of heart attack, high cholesterol, high blood pressure, diabetes, and some forms of cancer.[14]

You also burn calories when you do cardio. You may in fact burn more calories per minute than when you do strength training. However, muscle tissue burns more calories than fat tissue, so with strength training, you'll continue to burn calories even after you have completed your workout. Yes, even while you're at home sitting on the sofa watching Netflix.

Increasing your muscle mass is a key factor in weight loss. Period. If you want to become strong, see your body change, and still be able to eat while dropping fat, then resistance training should be your top priority. It will increase your metabolism, shape your body, reduce insulin sensitivity, and burn more total calories over time.

BUT I DON'T WANT TO BE BULKY

I know somewhere in your mind, there's a voice saying, "Ugh, but Sonia, I really don't want to look bulky!" Let me take a moment to say this in very clear English: You will *not* get bulky by lifting weights. You know those female bodybuilders who look really muscular? The ones who are strong but also pretty thick? Those women train, eat, and take supplements specifically to look like that. In fact, it takes years of dedication and commitment to achieve that kind of physique.

The reality is this: when you pick up heavy things, your muscles get stronger but not necessarily bigger. If you pump yourself full of testosterone and eat way more calories than you're burning every day while you lift heavy things? Then yes, you'll probably get bigger.

LIMITING BELIEF
Other women can lift weights, but if I do,
I'll start to look manly.

NEW BELIEF
I trust that resistance training is the most effective
way for me to achieve my goals. The more muscle I have, the
faster my metabolism will be, which is key to my success.

MORE IS NOT BETTER

Now that we've cleared that up, let's move on to how often you should be strength training. As you can imagine, there isn't a simple formula that's right for everyone. It all depends on what your goals and values are, how active you already are, and ultimately what feels realistic for you. Many people think they need to work out seven days a week to see results, but that's absolutely wrong. It's about tuning in to your body and listening to what it needs, rather than pushing to create a perfect daily routine. In fact, I have seen significantly better results in my own body when I'm working out three or four days a week than when I was working out seven days a week, often twice a day. Seriously, I've done all the experiments in this department, so let me save you the legwork (literally): more is not always better when it comes to fitness.

Never did I realize this more than when I was postpartum with my first child. It was a really tough time for me. I felt like I was juggling so many variables—navigating severe anxiety while troubleshooting the different phases of infanthood, surviving post-baby marriage, living with my parents while renovating our condo, and getting back into media. It was complicated, and the last thing on my mind was working out. It felt beyond my capacity. Like, I was doing so much "heavy lifting" mentally, I just couldn't stomach the idea of *literal* heavy lifting. It took me seven months to work up the mental endurance to go back to the gym—even though I was a "health and wellness expert" (what would people think?), even though I knew that exercise would make me feel better, even though I missed feeling strong both physically and mentally. God, it was intimidating and uncomfortable to go back to the gym after such a long hiatus. I felt like a foreigner in a place that used to be my happy home. It was daunting to think about how much fat I had gained and how much strength I had lost.

What if I couldn't do it?

What if my body had changed forever?

What if all my pretty workout clothes would never fit again?

And yet, there was a small part of me that was also excited about the challenge that lay ahead.

Slowly but surely, I navigated my way back to fitness. I focused on rebuilding my strength, tackled small wins at the gym, and concentrated on cleaning up my diet in the limited time I had. I had a lot on my plate, and the amount of time and energy I could give to working out was rather scant. Some weeks, I'd only work out at home because I couldn't stomach getting myself to the gym. Other weeks, I'd just do a couple of short spin sessions to keep me from spiraling both mentally and physically. Not a lot of effort, as you can see, and yet I got surprisingly positive results. Once I stopped beating my body into submission and started taking the "less is more" approach using weight lifting and HIIT (high-intensity interval training) over endless cardio and starvation, my body responded with, "Oh yes, now *this* is something I can get on board with. Forever."

The perfectionist in me could see that I didn't have to be so hardcore, working out six or seven days a week for ninety minutes at a time, to achieve the results that I wanted. I knew that overtraining was a thing, and when it came to working with my clients, I was always cognizant of that fact. But somehow, when it came to my own body, I had never been able to adopt the same principles. Before having my baby, I had put my body into overdrive mode thinking it was the price I had to pay to be lean and strong. Now, though, I was seeing the benefits of a saner approach.

And you can, too.

My recommendation is to strength train three or four days a week. There are a few ways to do this:

- Total body (same workout each time)
- Total body (alternating, focusing on either total-body pushing or pulling movements in each session)
- Upper/lower (alternating between focusing on either upper- or lower-body exercises each session)

WHAT'S WHAT AND WHERE?

The primary muscles in a "push workout" include the chest, triceps, quadriceps, calves, and shoulders. Examples of push exercises are push-ups, squats, and shoulder presses.

A "pull workout" is the exact opposite. Pull exercises are those where the muscles contract when weight is being pulled toward your body. The primary muscles in a pull workout include all back muscles, biceps, hamstrings, obliques, and the trapezius muscles. Examples of pull exercises are pull-ups, back rows, deadlifts, rear shoulder flys, and bicep curls.[15]

When it comes to what kind of strength training to do, I recommend that you focus on compound movements. These are exercises that utilize multiple joints at a time, like:

- Deadlifts
- Squats
- Push-ups
- Pull-ups
- Rows
- Dips

The majority of your workout should be made up of these sorts of movements because they recruit the largest amount of muscle tissue. This burns the most calories, which in turn burns the most fat over time.[16] You could also do tricep kickbacks and bicep curls, but look at the size of those muscle groups: they're relatively small. If you're trying to optimize your time and effort to get the quickest results, then working larger muscle groups like your chest, back, legs, and core will ensure you get the biggest bang for your buck.

THE BASICS

There are a few key terms to know as well:

- **Repetition (or rep).** A rep is one completion of an exercise, such as one deadlift, one bench press, or one arm curl.

- **Set.** A set is a series of repetitions performed sequentially. For example, eight repetitions can make up one set of bench presses.

- **Rest interval.** This is the time spent resting between sets to allow the muscle to recover. The rest period between sets usually ranges from thirty seconds to two minutes. Some exercises also have short or minor rests between reps.

- **Repetition maximum (or RM).** An RM is your personal best or the most you can lift once in a single repetition of an exercise. Therefore, a 12RM is the most you can lift while successfully performing twelve repetitions with proper form.

How many reps and sets should you be doing during your workouts? Is the perfect number six? Eight? Fifteen?

If you're just starting out, then my suggestion is to focus on maintaining pristine form and technique while mastering each exercise.[17] Perfectionists, rejoice! While "done is better than perfect" in life, when it comes to exercise, I'll say that perfect is crucial to get the most out of an exercise safely. Learning which muscles are being recruited during an exercise and perfecting proper technique is absolutely critical for a beginner. Proper technique will not only help you avoid injury, but also ensure that you're getting the most from each exercise. Forget about lifting weights that feel excruciatingly heavy and focus on weights that feel challenging but doable so that you can concentrate on emphasizing the muscle groups that are deliberately being worked in each exercise.

Here's what a session might look like for a beginner:

- Reps: ten to fifteen
- Weight: 60 to 70 percent of 1RM
- Sets: two to three
- Rest: thirty to sixty seconds between sets

This rep, set, and weight range is best if you are new to training or recovering from an injury. Training within this rep range will build strength, muscular endurance, coordination, and cardiovascular fitness without really growing muscle size. It will also prevent your nervous and muscular systems from going into shock as they deal with the new physical stimulus. Suddenly lifting heavy things regularly is a big adjustment for your body. As you get stronger week by week, you can slowly increase your weight and lower the number of reps you're doing, as long as you can maintain perfect technique.

As you gain experience, your workouts can start to change. Here's what a workout could look like for an intermediate who is looking to tone, sculpt, and increase their muscle:[18]

- Reps: eight to ten
- Weight: 75 to 90 percent of 1RM
- Sets: three to four
- Rest: forty-five to ninety seconds between sets

Remember, you won't get bulky; this will help you elevate your metabolism and build those curves. You'll want to make sure to include "periodization" into your workout routine. This means increasing or decreasing both the volume and intensity of your program so that your workouts don't become too routine. Once your body adapts to your program, it's important to tweak it so that you can keep your muscles guessing.

TO GYM OR NOT TO GYM?

A lot of people ask me which machines are best to use at the gym, but machines aren't ideal. They limit natural movement and recruit less muscle tissue, which in turn makes your workout kind of weak. Compound movements without a machine, on the other hand, will not only burn tons of calories during your workout but also keep you burning calories long after you're done. The exception to this is the cable machine. Whereas exercise machines tend to stabilize the body and isolate the muscles of a specific lift, cable exercises are typically performed standing, which means that your lower body and abs are always involved.

If you are new to all of this, let's be clear about one thing: you don't have to muster up the courage or energy to go to the gym.

I'll say it again: *you don't have to go to the gym to get fit.*

There's plenty that you can do in the comfort of your own home to rev up your metabolism, build some muscle, and burn fat. In terms of compound movements, you can pretty much do all the necessary ones without any equipment: squats, lunges, step-ups, burpees, planks, push-ups, supermans, and more.

LIMITING BELIEF
*I have to go to the gym to be dedicated
to my health and wellness.*

NEW BELIEF
Fitness is a priority in my life regardless of where and when I choose to work out. I trust that I can be flexible with my workout schedule without falling off the wagon.

HIIT (HIGH-INTENSITY INTERVAL TRAINING)

You can also use HIIT to push yourself to the max without weights.[19] HIIT is a broad term for workouts that involve short periods of intense exercise alternated with recovery periods. One of the biggest advantages of HIIT is that you can get maximal health benefits in minimal time. This is particularly effective for those of you who value living your life over spending long periods of time working out.

My favorite form of HIIT is Tabata, inspired by Dr. Izumi Tabata, in which you do twenty seconds of max intensity exercise followed by ten seconds of rest, repeated eight times for a total of four minutes.[20] That's it: four minutes. There's no way you can tell me that you don't have four minutes to spare in your day. Don't lie.

Burpees, jump squats, push-ups, mountain climbers, and deadlifts are all great exercises to do interval-style. They all blast large muscle groups in one shot. If I'm tight on time, I'll do a four-minute burpee sequence and call that my workout for the day. If I have more time or I'm in the mood for a longer workout, then I'll often pair multiple interval sets, each focusing on different muscle groups. For example:

- Legs: jump squats, four minutes, Tabata style
- Rest one minute
- Chest: push-ups, four minutes, Tabata style
- Rest one minute
- Back: rows, four minutes, Tabata style
- Rest one minute
- Core: planks, four minutes, Tabata style

Done! Total workout time: twenty minutes.

Now let's talk about effort. A lot of people go to the gym, but once they're there, they just coast along, doing what feels easy. How many people have you seen bobbing up and down on the elliptical reading a magazine or talking on the phone? Seriously, it's infuriating. If you can read a book while doing cardio, you can essentially assume you aren't going to be reaping any dramatic benefits from your session other than "active recovery." Sure, *something* is always better than nothing, but real progress requires *real* work. More often than not, it should feel challenging, and if it doesn't, you need to push yourself until it does.

When doing any interval training, it's important that you train to exhaustion. You should have nothing left to give at the end of an exercise. Your muscles should be totally out of commission within the twenty- or thirty-second interval that you're doing. If you can squeeze in even one more rep, then you should aim to increase your load or push yourself to work harder and faster. The idea is to push your muscles hard to max them out. You should be breathing heavily, your heart rate should be up, and your muscles should feel exhausted when you are done.

The saying is lame, but it really is true: all progress comes from going outside your comfort zone.

JUST GET IT DONE

It's important to get out of your comfort zone and force yourself to work out for even just a week. If you're exercising in the comfort of your own home, then get yourself the equipment you need to play around with different exercises. Some of my favorite at-home workout tools include:

- gliders
- TRX straps
- all-in-one dumbbells
- Bosu ball
- stability ball
- resistance bands
- yoga mat

If you have a gym membership, I bet you'll find that the super-scary weights area with the super-scary-looking people isn't all that bad. In fact, I bet that you'll start to enjoy learning and trying new things. You just have to be willing to take the first bold step and put yourself out there.

YOU'D BETTER *WERK*

There is one key factor to a successful workout regimen: showing up.

When you're committing to a workout plan, *do it.*

Even if you're (kind of) tired, even if it's (sort of) cold outside, even if you're not (really) in the mood. This is where we practice living our mindset shifts. This is where we practice showing up for what *really matters*. This is where we practice commitment, resilience, and tenacity to claim agency over our journey.

It's going to get tough. It always does. There will be days when you feel like it's just not worth the effort, but this is when you'll refine the process of showing up for yourself using the tools you have available to you. Assess and evaluate where the "fatigue" really is. Is it in your mind or your body? Do you *really* need rest (it's okay if you do), or are you slowly playing to the beat of your limiting beliefs and perfectionist tendencies again? Reconnect with your values. Reflect on your Mindset Manifesto. Effort and consistency are key.

My personal suggestion? Don't let more than three days go by without a workout unless you're deliberately taking a week off for rest and recovery. Seriously, if I don't work out for three days, it's really easy for me to make that the whole week, which can easily turn into a month (depending on how far into the current month I already am), which can easily turn into a quarter, which can turn into an entire season, and then before I know it, I'm in a year-long rut. Get to know yourself. Figure out your personal threshold. Remember, exercise isn't always going to feel easy. In fact, most of the time it won't.

What parameters do *you* need to put in place to ensure you're living in alignment with your values?

To ensure that you show up even when you don't want to?

To keep yourself firmly in the driver's seat, even when the road starts to get a little bumpy?

REFLECT AND REMEMBER

Reflect

How might shifting your focus from how you look to *what feels good* change your approach to fitness? When you strip away the limiting beliefs and external noise, what feels most authentic to you?

Remember

1. Strength training is the most effective form of exercise for fat loss. Building muscle will boost your metabolism, sculpt your body, reduce insulin sensitivity, and burn more total calories over time.

2. You do not have to go to the gym to get fit. Plain and simple. If it doesn't work for you, don't do it.

3. *Showing up* is the one key factor to a successful workout regimen. It will get tough. Claim agency over your journey and practice commitment and resilience.

13
What Do You Really Want?

NOW THAT YOUR TOOLKIT IS well-equipped with the fundamentals of fitness and nutrition, I hope that you're feeling empowered to take aligned, tangible steps toward *real* change.

I know we've spent a lot of time talking about how to avoid blindly conquering arbitrary health and wellness goals. You get it. You know that path leads to nowhere. You know it's what keeps you stuck on the hamster wheel of weight loss. But now we've come to the point in the journey where you actually *do* have to get clear on your goals in order to give you the long-term vision and short-term motivation you need. This is where you break down your values and create a road map to further focus your knowledge, organize your time and resources, and get into the driver's seat of your life.

PRIORITIES MATTER

It's crucial that you clarify what you *really* want based on the values you established earlier in this book, and then set goals based on those priorities. Ask yourself questions like:

- Am I motivated to lose fat?
- Do I want to build muscle?
- Is feeling energetic important to me?

One of my clients spent years of her life spinning in circles because she was trying her best to gain muscle and lose fat at the same time. She thought she wanted both, so she spent her time lifting heavy weights while maintaining a severe caloric deficit to achieve lightning-speed results.

Unfortunately, most people can't lose fat and build muscle at the same time by following a conventional diet plan that has them severely restricting their calories. I say "most people" because some people can and do build a decent amount of muscle while they're in a caloric deficit, but that phenomenon is generally limited to people who are very overweight and have never lifted weights before, or those who are returning to exercise after a long break, where muscle memory comes into play. But in general? No. It can't really be done. To lose fat, you must be in a caloric deficit. And to gain muscle, you typically need a caloric surplus.

Let me say it again: *You need a caloric deficit to lose weight. You need a caloric surplus to gain muscle.*

My client was driving herself nuts for years, getting on and falling off the wagon time and time again. It wasn't until she and I cleared up the confusion and got laser-focused on her priorities that she saw the results she truly wanted. By overhauling her workout regimen—reducing her workouts from seven days a week to four days a week—and focusing on alternate periods of negative calorie balance with periods of positive calorie balance, we achieved the results she had always wanted within a year.

SMARTEN UP

It can be a real challenge to drown out the noise that's constantly pushing and pulling us in different directions. We're so heavily influenced by what others expect of us, what we're told we're *supposed* to care about, and what we see online, that we struggle to stay aligned with our purpose and priorities.

What should your goals be? That's absolutely personal and depends on what you want.

Really: *What do you actually want?*

When we set goals that are informed by what's most important to us, we're able to take action that no longer feels soul-sucking. I've always been the master of achieving goals—what I set my mind to, I achieve, no matter how painful. But as you know, I've also had a pattern of climbing to the tops of mountains only to look around and say, "Oh shit, I thought happiness lived up here, but all I'm actually feeling is anxiety about where to go next." Remember those shape-shifting goals we talked about earlier? Guilty. My target was always moving, my goals always morphing, so I was never able to *feel* a sense of accomplishment. However, when I started to set concrete, realistic, achievable goals that were *actually* aligned with my core values, I was able to stop spinning myself in circles, experiencing real progress and satisfaction along the way.

This is where I like to bring in SMART goals. These are:

Specific

Measurable

Attainable

Relevant

Time sensitive

I know, the concept of SMART goals is pretty Business 101. There's nothing revolutionary about what I'm suggesting here. We all know we should set goals. We all know they shouldn't be random and vague.

And yet . . . how many times have you vowed to "start again" by simply saying:

- "Tomorrow I'm going to eat healthier and really stick to it."
- "On Monday I'm going to start going to the gym again."
- "Next week I'm going to get my shit together and get back into a routine."

Vague AF, am I right? Like, what does any of this *really* mean? How are you supposed to progress when you don't have something concrete to build a strategy around?

Establishing both short-term and long-term SMART goals sets the tone for your journey, allowing you to stay focused and helping you override your negative narrative. You move away from the ever-changing goal of "skinny" and begin working toward something concrete. You also have something tangible to benchmark yourself against, which enables you to course-correct at every turn. It's a simple mechanism, but it's *so* powerful.

Here's an example of a short-term goal that my clients and I have set: "I want to lose three inches from my waist in the next three months."

Here's an example of a long-term goal: "I want to lose twenty inches head to toe by the end of the year."

As you can see, I like to pick goals that relate to size, not weight, because we all know the scale is a lying, cheating bastard. In addition to picking size-related goals, I also mandate that my clients establish performance-oriented goals. For example, "In the short term, I want to be able to hold a plank for one minute. In the long term, I want to be able to do twenty-five push-ups without taking a break in between." Or . . . "I want to run a half-marathon." Or . . . "I want to climb Machu Picchu." If you have no interest in working out, a performance goal can be as simple as "I want to eat three salads a week to make sure I'm getting more vegetables in my diet." These performance-based goals shift the focus from size to strength.

From skinny to healthy.

From aesthetics to wellness.

Take it from me: once you start to see progress in the health department, you'll start to care less and less about the size department. Once you can do twenty-five push-ups, you'll be like, "Holy shit, I'm kind of amazing! If I can do twenty-five, what's stopping me from doing thirty? Fifty?" You'll want to eat for performance, sleep for performance, and hydrate for performance. Seriously, it wasn't until I stopped obsessing over my size and started focusing on my athletic performance that I felt a shift. I started to marvel at my potential. I started to appreciate my capacity. I started to *love* my body.

REAL PROGRESS TAKES REAL TIME

Now, a quick word of caution, because if you're not vigilant, you'll likely get impatient and slip back into old patterns—getting caught up in external noise, playing the comparison game, and disconnecting from your sense of agency.

We're human. It happens to the best of us.

You see, goals make us feel productive, but when we're not *really* tuned in, we end up once again racing toward the "end destination," ignoring all the data and feedback our bodies are trying to share with us along the way. We miss the opportunities to course-correct our mindset and actions because we're "in it to win it," not realizing that we're slowly slipping away from how we want to *feel*. Before we know it, the whole system breaks.

It's just so easy to fall into the "am I skinny yet" trap two weeks into your new regimen no matter how committed you are to slow and steady progress. The rational part of you understands that results take time, but our environments have conditioned us to expect visible results ASAP. Don't be fooled by the glossy content you see showcasing people "crushing their wellness goals"—it's a lot harder than it looks. The #hashtag world makes us question ourselves and preys on our insecurities, but you know as well as I do that there's no such thing as "Eight Simple Hacks to Build Muscle" or a "One-Week Workout for Visible Abs." Maintaining steady progress takes time and commitment. There is no linear path to success. Remember what we talked about earlier? This time, it's about progress, not perfection. This is going to be an iterative process. It's going to take time to collect the data. It's going to take time to refine your habits and behaviors. It's going to take time for your body to start responding to all these new stimuli. Accepting the process is the only way to progress.

Embrace the work instead of hoping for a miracle fix. Ground your actions in your core values. Give yourself a real chance to form positive habits and resolve not to give up two weeks later when "nothing is happening." Evaluate your progress week over week and ask yourself, "Am I getting stronger? Do I feel better?" Week over week, the answer should be clear and positive. If it's not, then don't be afraid to tweak the system. Somewhere along the way, as the weeks pass by, I know you'll start to see that this shift in both your mindset and your approach to fitness will improve your life forever.

REFLECT AND REMEMBER

Reflect

What do you really want? Is there anything holding you back from writing it down? What fears come up, if any? Are you challenging yourself to connect with the real you?

Remember

1. You need to clarify your priorities because it's impossible to accomplish everything at the same time. Be honest with yourself about what you *really* want to achieve beyond the obvious "I want to feel better" statements you already know.

2. Setting SMART goals is an effective way to keep yourself motivated, focused, and balanced as you navigate the ebbs and flows of your health and wellness journey.

3. Tune in. It's so easy to get caught up in old patterns, chasing an "end destination" and losing sight of what really matters. Throughout your journey give yourself gentle reminders of what you're working toward and how you want to feel so that you don't get caught up in other, more destructive emotions.

14

Choosing the Unknown

NOW, I KNOW YOU MAY be feeling pretty pumped to map out your new and improved wellness regimen based on your clear, crisp goals. I get it. Goals feel actionable. They make us feel charged up. They make us feel like we can get into "doing mode." We *love* goals.

But how do we make sure that we're *really* setting ourselves up for success and happiness this time around? Notice how I added "happiness" into the equation? Success is synonymous with achieving our goals. Happiness, on the other hand, comes when we're able to find joy *in the journey* toward achieving our goals. When we strive for success, we often do so at the expense of everything else, abandoning our Mindset Manifesto, playing the comparison game, doing whatever it takes to "get there" as fast as possible because that's where happiness awaits.

I know this all too well.

I was twenty-one years old, finishing up my degree with all the right ticky marks. I was engaged to an older guy who met all the parental criteria. I'd soon be starting what I believed was my "dream job" as a corporate executive. And I was considered brown-girl beautiful—long hair, fair skin, thin body (thanks to my disordered eating habits), and thin eyebrows (thanks to my Revlon tweezers). Yes, I had made it to the "end destination" and was only months away from checking marriage off my "happiness to-do list."

But as I got closer to the wedding, my princess-cut engagement ring started to feel less like a flawless diamond and more like a glass box that I was being held hostage in. I had just started to settle into my own skin, and the more I did, the less my reality made sense to me. How had I gotten here? How had I been so tuned in to the voices of other people? How had I not seen that I'd never really been happy? Too busy suppressing, compressing, and denying parts of myself in order to achieve success and stay in my relationship.

Holy shit. What had I done?

It made me sick to my stomach, but I broke the news to my parents: I don't think I can go through with the wedding.

And in that moment, I broke their hearts.

I was shattered. You see, I grew up in what some may consider your typical Indian household, where high performance was the norm, image was everything, and feelings were swept under the Persian rug. As expected, my parents were viscerally against me calling off my wedding.

I mean, what would people think? How could I, their daughter, do something like this? And how would I ever recover from the guilt of ruining everyone's lives?

Total chaos ensued.

I was two weeks out from my first wedding event. All my family from India had already arrived. And there I was, backed into a corner, having a literal panic attack on my bathroom floor.

I felt trapped by the shame of it all.

It felt too early for me to be making "the biggest mistake of my life." But which choice would be the biggest mistake? Following through with the wedding because this was all I'd ever been taught, or calling it off and facing the unknown?

I chose the unknown. And the unknown was me.

This one decision changed the entire course of my life. I broke free from the pressure to try and fit into the perfect mold, which allowed me to hear the faint whisper of my soul, the voice that was saying, "Break free, little one, jump out of the car; you'll find your way."

Everything changed from there. By tuning in to who I really was, I could begin living a life guided by *my* internal compass. My voice. Not what had been projected on me through my culture, and my parents, and the random aunties who always have opinions about everyone's lives except their own. You know which aunties I'm talking about.

Everyone expects a moment of clarity. But for me, it was a messy, messy chapter. Therapy. Journaling. Breathwork. Tears. And honest and uncomfortable conversations with others and myself.

Through it all . . . I found freedom.

The freedom to trust myself.

The freedom to explore what I wanted and needed.

The freedom to finally be "enough," exactly where I was, instead of speeding toward the "end destination."

HAPPINESS STARTS NOW

You know as well as I do that there is no "You Are Happy Now" trophy waiting for you at the finish line, no matter what goal you achieve. It's about finding joy in the journey—each triumph and setback teaching us more about who we are and what we want, allowing us the opportunity to course-correct and refine what isn't working. It's about curiosity, learning, and growing every step of the way in order to achieve your potential.

Happiness is just like anything else: If you're not making shifts toward happiness *now*, it's not going to come later, no matter how much you achieve. You actually have to practice it, like a skill, so that you can get better at it. Sounds bizarre, I know. But it's kind of the same way you don't just magically clean up your diet or conquer your new workout routine in one day. It takes time to refine your ability to do these things consistently without falling off the wagon. It takes patience to stay the course until these things become second nature. Happiness is no different. You actually have to *try* to cultivate it today so that you can experience it more tomorrow.

It wasn't until I began to look at the concept of happiness as a "practice" instead of a "natural state of being" that I started to shift how I was showing up in my life. Instead of waiting for happiness to strike, I started looking for opportunities to be curious, taking pleasure in collecting feedback wherever I could.

"Oh hey, I'm experiencing momentum and I'm on track to achieve my goals. This feels amazing!"

What is working? How can I replicate this in the future? How can I maintain my stride?

"Ugh, I'm feeling stuck, overwhelmed, like I keep taking two steps forward, one step back."

Why? What can I learn from this? How can I shift my behaviors and actions? How can I effect change?

It all comes back to abandoning the idea of the "end destination" and learning to enjoy the ride, no matter how bumpy the road gets. It's all insight. It's all feedback. It's all *for* you.

REFLECT AND REMEMBER

Reflect

Are you still waiting to reach an imaginary end goal instead of refocusing your energy on creating joy throughout your journey?

Remember

1. Happiness is not a product of success. Instead, happiness is what keeps us motivated as we work toward achieving our goals.

2. Look for opportunities to be curious, take pleasure in collecting feedback, and find joy in the journey.

3. Stop holding out for a later moment that may never come instead of appreciating what's right in front of you. Happiness begins today.

15

Know Thyself

WE KNOW THAT GOING AFTER the same thing with the same actions and hoping for a different result means that we're living in a dream world. If we want real, long-lasting results this time around, *something* needs to be different.

What is that something going to be? How are you going to make sure that this time around, you're setting yourself up for success? That you're moving in alignment with your values?

It's important that you understand the value of tuning in to your body. You can't solve a problem if you don't know what it is, and your body is constantly trying to give you messages about what kinds of tweaks it needs. The problem is, we rarely pause to listen. We're so busy trying to get on with fixing problems that we fail to stop and connect with ourselves to better focus our efforts.

SELF-CARE (JUST FOR YOU)

When you're moving a mile a minute, it's so easy to miss the signals and messages your mind and body are trying to share with you. But these messages hold so much insight that can support you on your journey. The tricky part is tuning in.

I'll admit that when I'm focused on conquering my to-do list, I rarely pause to ask myself how I'm feeling. So, my first simple suggestion? Practice taking a break. Whether it's through a few minutes of meditation, breathwork, light stretching, or simply going for a short walk, learning to slow down is the first step to being able to tune in to how your mind and body are feeling. And no, this doesn't include numbing yourself on the sofa with Netflix or mindlessly scrolling your Instagram feed after a long day at work, because while you may feel like that's the easiest version of slowing down, it doesn't facilitate your ability to look inward.

Self-care is good for the mind, body, and soul. It's such a common buzzword these days that we're all like, "No shit, obviously it's good to care about yourself." But what is self-care, really? And why is it considered so crucial?

Contrary to popular belief, the point of self-care isn't to tick things off an indulgent list of to-dos. It has nothing to do with taking hour-long baths or getting regular massages (although let's be real, I'm all for massages). Rather, self-care is just a commitment to doing whatever it takes to care for ourselves physically, mentally, and emotionally over the long term. Committing to self-care takes a bit of time and effort, but it's well worth it, given that self-care supports:

- **Better productivity.** When you learn to make time for the things that support your health and well-being and say no to things that overextend you, you can slow down, recenter, and focus better.

- **Better physical health.** When you understand that stress can take a serious toll on your body—it can weaken your immune system and leave you feeling defeated—you give your body a real opportunity to heal and recover.

- **Enhanced self-esteem.** When you regularly carve out time to be good to yourself and meet your own needs, you send a positive message to your brain that you matter, which can greatly reduce negative self-talk.

You don't have to pick anything extravagant to add to your daily self-care list to do it right. Taking a warm shower, making a cup of your favorite tea (without multitasking), or writing in a journal can do wonders. Self-care doesn't have to sound cool or be Insta-worthy to be effective. The point is to prioritize yourself and your needs. The more you do, the better you'll be able to grow, thrive, and connect with yourself.

LET YOUR BODY TALK

Once you've gotten into the rhythm of your self-care practice, you may want to incorporate some version of a body scan into your weekly regimen. I personally like to do this every week when I'm reflecting on my Mindset Manifesto. It helps me deepen the connection between my body and mind. It helps me remember that I'm not just living from the neck up. It helps me evaluate how I'm really feeling and what I actually need.

The point of a body scan is to focus your attention on different parts of your body, all the way from the muscles in your face down to your feet. This may sound like a lot of work, but a body scan is just a simple relaxation technique that can enhance your ability to explore and just "be" with your body. Here's what you do:

- Lie down on a comfortable surface and close your eyes.

- Be aware of your breath and begin to intentionally relax.

- Start with your toes and work your way up to your ankles, your legs, your knees, your hips, your belly, your back, your shoulders, your neck, your eyes, and finally your head.

- Think about each part of your body and consider how it's feeling. What observations can you make? Does anything feel not quite right? Do you feel pain, discomfort, or angst around any specific area of your body? What thoughts come up about your body and your health?

- Grab a journal or a scrap piece of paper and write down anything you feel like capturing. How did you feel physiologically during and after the practice?

- Notice any feelings or emotions that come up. Instead of glossing over sensations or emotions, try to be curious and ask why. The point is to get used to connecting with your body so you can do it more easily and readily in day-to-day life.

It wasn't until I began to tune in to what my body was trying to tell me that I started to feel like I was breaking my lifelong cycle of defeat.

"Am I dehydrated?"

"Do I need more sleep?"

"How many days a week do I need to work out to see progress? How many days will lead to burnout?"

Tuning in to my body and exploring questions like these allowed me to course-correct my mindset and behaviors. I started to pay attention to the sensations in my body, like whether I was perpetually "headachey" or thirsty or fatigued. I began to observe how my body responded to stimuli like low-carb diets versus high-fat diets, or strength training versus cardio. And along with all this, I started to layer positivity into my life, from mindfulness to basic meditation to stress management techniques. It wasn't an overnight thing but rather a steady process of slowing down and looking inward to ensure my actions were aligned with my goals.

Now here's the ironic part of it all. Not until I started focusing on my *overall wellness*, instead of my size, did I ultimately achieve the body I had always pined for. I was strong. I was lean. I had all kinds of definition. And I was proud because instead of taking an easy detour, I had fought through the mess and come out the other side a different person.

REFLECT AND REMEMBER

Reflect

Are you ready to layer self-care into your daily or weekly practice? What barriers come up for you when you think about prioritizing "me time"?

Remember

1. Your body knows what it needs. The trick is slowing down and shutting out the noise so that you can hear what it's trying to tell you.

2. Your version of self-care is for you and you alone. Nothing has to be fancy or complicated; the goal is to simply slow down and listen to the messages your mind and body are trying to give you.

3. Strive to develop a sense of curiosity about how you and your body are feeling. This will help you create a health and wellness regimen that feels aligned with yourself and your values.

16

Celebrate Yourself
(... It's Actually Important)

NOW, IF YOU'RE ANYTHING LIKE me, you're probably not a natural at "self-celebration." As you know, I was raised by strict Indian parents—we didn't celebrate anything, ever, because there was always something greater to be achieved. But as an adult, I'm happy to say that self-celebration is something I'm working on, and I encourage you to take a stab at it, too. I mean, why shouldn't we pat ourselves on the back for the progress we're making?

We're showing up.

We're doing the things.

We're seeing the impact.

It all deserves acknowledgment and celebration, and frankly it makes the journey a lot less painful.

NEW TOOLS FOR A NEW NARRATIVE

When we talk about practicing happiness, it doesn't require much to make the shift. A few simple tools can really help reorient our narrative from negative to positive.

From perfection to progress.

From the "end destination" to the journey.

TRACK YOUR PROGRESS

I use a large calendar to reflect my week-over-week progress and momentum. I know this sounds a little elementary, but trust me, it works. We *all* like gold stars—we have since primary school. I give my daughter a gold star sticker every time she demonstrates qualities like bravery, integrity, and compassion. I give my son a gold star sticker every time he successfully goes pee in the toilet. And I give myself a gold star sticker for each day that I work out, eat according to my goals, and practice self-care so that I can pat myself on the back and say, "Hey, Sonia, you're nailing this whole 'claiming your own agency' thing." Don't like stickers? Then find some kind of progress tracker, something that makes you feel excited when you look at it and that you can keep updated easily. I've tried a bunch of apps that have been finicky and complicated, so I stick with the old-school methods, but play around with what works for you. If it's a pain in the ass, you won't do it, you'll feel stressed and behind, and (speaking from experience) you'll likely end up eating pizza and crying. Let's avoid that.

TREAT YO'SELF

For some people, a treat can be as simple as a delicious warm brownie. For others, it's new fitness apparel or the latest tech gadget. Regardless of what you choose, the point is to celebrate when you conquer a milestone. Hit thirty days of following your routine? Treat yo'self! Managed to pack your lunch every day for two weeks? Treat yo'self! These treats don't need to be big; they just need to feel like a moment of acknowledgment. A moment of positive reinforcement. A moment to say, "I'm proud of myself." You may not be anywhere close to achieving your short- or long-term goals, but you're acknowledging the fact that you're showing up for yourself, and *that* makes the journey worthwhile. Some people I know also use the concept of treats to keep themselves accountable during their journey. For instance, one of my clients puts two dollars in a mason jar every time she goes to the gym. She sets a dollar target for herself in advance, and then once she hits that target, she takes out the money and gets a facial. Like, how brilliant is that. She works out while also supporting her "facial fund."

LEAN ON AFFIRMATIONS

I love affirmations. In fact, I practice them every morning: just a few basic phrases that I say quietly to myself to start my day on the right foot. They ensure that I'm centered, in tune, and ready to tackle the day with intention as opposed to letting the day take hold of me. Examples of affirmations that work for me are:

- "I am healthy, energetic, and optimistic."
- "I trust my body to know what it needs, and I listen."
- "My body is healing and I feel better every day."

And sometimes...

- "I am clear and in control, like a really good deodorant."

Essentially, affirmations are positive self-statements that, if repeated over time, convince you that they are true. By extension, affirmations boost your self-esteem and problem-solving skills. It has been shown that people under high levels of stress can foster better problem-solving and decision-making skills just by reinforcing what is important to them on a regular basis.[21] With affirmations, you're essentially training your mind to think differently. You're overriding the negative self-talk. You're preemptively finding rebuttal arguments for the negative voices in your head.

FIND YOUR PERSON

Find an accountability partner, someone to keep you on track when it's minus-forty degrees outside and you don't want to get out of bed at 5 a.m. to work out. We get tired, we get cold, we get sick, we get stressed, and we "just don't want to" after a while. Finding someone who can be on the journey with us means that we don't have to constantly be the one to pep ourselves up. This person can be your spouse, your best friend, a colleague, or a workout buddy. It doesn't matter whether or not you're actually working out with the person; all that matters is that they know you have real goals to attain, and they are committed to giving you a gentle (or firm) slap in the face, should you need it. And yes, ultimately, we all need it. Be specific with your accountability buddy and schedule a weekly call or check-in if it isn't someone you see regularly. Even if you do see them regularly, it's still a good idea to debrief every couple of weeks just to vent and course-correct. Also, take it upon yourself to become someone else's accountability partner—you may be the missing piece in someone else's journey.

SELF-LOVE LANGUAGE

There's no obligation to use all (or any) of the tools that I've suggested. What works for me may not work for you, so keep exploring, modifying, and recalibrating until you find an effective personal system. Finding what works for you is a tender, loving process—take your time with it, make it a phase of gentle exploration.

We've all heard about love languages: the different ways in which individuals give and receive love. Maybe you've spent hours (like me) trying to figure out how you express and experience love in your external relationships. But have you thought about love languages in the context of your relationship with *yourself*?

Are you someone who needs positive self-statements to feel like you're being treated well?

Are you someone who needs to acknowledge themselves with a purchase (or "gift")?

Are you someone who needs to experience quality alone time to feel like you're honoring your needs?

Getting clear on your own self-love language will help you find the right tools for you to use as you reorient your focus from the "end destination" to the journey. Give yourself permission to show up for yourself. Look inward and listen—*really listen*—to what you need to feel celebrated. To feel rewarded. To feel like you are making progress. Your body and mind will tell you what they need. The data you collect will show you what works and what doesn't. You just need to commit to listening attentively, empathizing, and responding with a whole lot of self-love.

A BUMPY ROAD WELL TRAVELED

Your journey will never be linear. There will be high points, low points, and some surprise U-turns along the way. This is okay. This is normal. When it feels like you're getting sucked into the vortex again, don't panic. Instead, remind yourself of what *really* matters, of what you *really* want. Feeling stuck is not a sign that you're falling off the wagon. It's a sign that you need to reconnect with yourself so that you can prioritize how you feel over the noise that's telling you to focus on anything and everything else.

What if you were to use these moments of uncertainty to get to know yourself a little better?

What if in the spaces between achievements, like when you plateau or fall off the wagon, you were to learn new things about who you really are and what you really want out of life?

What if you were to use all this data to redefine how you intend to show up for yourself?

We are all works in progress. Do your best to release the negative self-talk and instead focus on replacing your inner narrative with statements that feel supportive, kind, and loving. Remember your Mindset Manifesto? Return to this touchstone whenever you start to feel like you're losing your way. This isn't going to be an overnight fix, and your Mindset Manifesto will remind you of your *why* whenever you feel like you're slipping away from who you want to be.

REFLECT AND REMEMBER

Reflect

Are you still struggling to celebrate yourself? Why are you struggling to show up for yourself in this way? What's holding you back?

Remember

1. Commit to celebrating your success to ground yourself in reality and build a sense of positive momentum.

2. Use whatever self-celebration tools work best to help you feel aligned with your wellness vision and get into the habit of practicing them regularly.

3. Progress is never linear. Return to your core values, evaluation criteria, and Mindset Manifesto whenever you feel out of alignment with your authenticity.

17

You Are the Driver

SO HERE WE ARE, AT the final stage of our journey together. We've gone from mind to body and back again, arriving at this new beginning for you. You now know just how crucial it is to get clear on your personal evaluation criteria in order to establish goals that are driven by what's most important to you. This is what will guide your future choices, behaviors, and actions. You now understand the cycle of limiting beliefs and can see how vital it is that you find a new, supportive narrative in order to overcome self-sabotage. This is what will set the stage for new possibilities, fresh motivation, and unwavering commitment. You're now clear on how perfectionism is holding you back and how necessary it is to abandon the idea of the "end destination" in order to practice happiness. This is what will shift how you feel about your body and your life. This is how you'll find happiness *today.*

THE *REAL* YOU

Looking back at my own journey, it's easy for me to see things clearly. Hindsight is always twenty-twenty. At the time, though, I had no idea what was simmering beneath the surface. I had no idea that somewhere in the dark corners of my brain lay this belief that happiness was merely ten pounds away, that I was living with this constant idea that "as soon as I look the way I want to, I'll arrive at happiness." I had no idea how much I attached my self-worth to my size. I had no idea how destructive my inner voice was. I had no idea how deeply I feared being average. I had no idea how desperately I wanted to prove my worth to myself, my parents, and the world. I had no idea how truly ugly I often felt in my skin. I had no idea how badly I wanted to see myself as successful. I had no idea how desperately I wanted to feel like I was "good enough."

When I look back at my quest to be thin, I'm now able to see it for what it really was. The negativity, the angst, the quiet panic, the constant negative or self-sabotaging inner dialogue: it was self-hate disguised as so many other things.

My transformation began the moment I felt I *deserved* better than being stuck on the hamster wheel of weight loss all my life. The moment I *believed* that there was a different path forward. The moment I *decided* enough was enough. My journey involved a lot of letting go. I had to let go of the idea that an Indian woman needs to have long hair to be considered beautiful. I had to let go of the idea that I needed to have a high-paying corporate career to be deemed intelligent and successful. I had to let go of all that my parents had taught me about happiness, this idea that getting all the ticky marks would lead to true contentment. I was done with it all. I was done with the façade. I said to hell with frailty (and my hair and my job). I wanted to *feel* strong. I wanted to *be* healthy. I wanted to *know* that I was being true to who I really am. And that's where the heavy lifting began, both figuratively and literally. I explored my values, dissected my limiting beliefs, abandoned the pursuit of perfection, and through it all found change, evolution, and progress. Day after day, week after week, I began to recognize the woman looking back at me in the mirror. Each time, she felt more and more like the *real* Sonia.

Now, it's your turn to come back to who *you* really are.

To shut out the noise.

To get clear.

To take aligned action.

THE PATH FORWARD

Before you dive headfirst into tracking your calories, lifting heavy things, and drinking more water, let me just take a quick moment to remind you that this is going to be an ongoing, iterative process. As much as it sucks to hear, I'm going to say it: you are not going to just read this book once, reconfigure your mindset, block out the #hashtag world, find a seamless new fitness and nutrition regimen, and quickly arrive at your ideal body.

You *will* experience setbacks and pitfalls. You will come up against feelings of negativity and frustration and defeat. You will have to find ways to dig yourself out of ruts and overcome plateaus. You will fall off the wagon. But also . . .

You *will* learn and grow throughout the journey.

You *will* find that the process gets easier and more enjoyable each step of the way.

You *will* see that "getting back on the wagon" no longer feels as difficult.

You *will* find that the struggle for motivation, dedication, and consistency begins to evaporate.

You *will* start to feel more confident and aligned with your "real" self.

You *will* experience more and more self-love.

You *will* begin to feel like you can embrace and celebrate change.

You *will* feel like you're worth it.

I know how good it feels to finally break free from all the angst, drama, and lies you've been telling yourself for so many years. The journey you're about to embark on is going to be both amazing and complicated. But mostly amazing. Yes, you're still going to struggle at times, but remember, you don't have to tackle everything at the same time, and you don't have to go through it alone. Falling off the wagon *is* going to happen. Because you're human. And because you're no longer going to expect and demand perfection from yourself. Don't panic: you can always pick up this book again and give yourself the reminders you need to recommit, refocus, and realign. When you start to feel like you're getting lost again, come back to this page and remind yourself of these three fundamentals.

A BODY YOU LOVE ISN'T WORTH A LIFE YOU HATE

When you take a step back from the "am I skinny yet?" narrative, you tune in to what you *really* need to achieve your health and wellness goals. By establishing core values (that are yours, and yours alone), you create a blueprint for your mindset that will carry you throughout your journey. Your Mindset Manifesto acts as the articulation, expression, and living touchstone of your values. Come back to your Manifesto every time you're tempted to try the latest TikTok "quick fix." Reflect on your Manifesto every time you find yourself taking action that feels kind of shitty. Sit with your Manifesto to bring you back to who you are every time you feel like the noise of the #hashtag world is getting too loud.

The external noise *will* get loud, which is why it's so crucial for you to confront and rewrite your inner narrative. Your limiting beliefs hold you back from achieving your goals, keeping you stuck in a failure loop that feels relentless. By letting go of self-judgment and discerning fact from fiction, you're able to establish a purposeful narrative that feels kind and supportive. When you stop being an asshole to yourself, you open the doors of limitless possibility and come one step closer to breaking your on-again, off-again cycle.

MOVE YOUR WAY TO A NEW MINDSET

Moving from your mind to your body is the first place to start manifesting your new mindset. It's how you claim agency over your life. It's how you start practicing and refining your thoughts, choices, and behaviors. It's how you see the power of your commitment, action, and resilience. When you claim agency over your life, making decisions no longer feels as heavy because you understand that you can't keep doing what you're doing, simply hoping for a different outcome.

The "mind work" and the "body work" always go hand in hand. This is how you connect your actions to your goals and your goals to your values. This is where you move away from the approach you're so used to and ground your actions in what *feels* good to you. Mindset without movement is just an intention, and action without intention is aimless. The two mutually reinforcing approaches help you break old patterns, refine your new way of living, and create a sense of *real* momentum.

THERE IS NO END DESTINATION

Happiness is not ten pounds away.

There is no "You Are Happy Now" trophy waiting for you at the finish line.

The "end destination" doesn't exist, no matter what the #hashtag world has you believe.

When you allow yourself the freedom to be "enough" exactly where you are instead of speeding toward the finish line, you find happiness *in* the journey. Each triumph feels like a beautiful step in the right direction. Each setback feels like an opportunity to collect feedback, refine, and course-correct your mindset and behaviors. By embracing curiosity, learning, and growth, instead of doing whatever it takes to get "there" faster, you enjoy the ride, no matter how bumpy the road gets. This is how you finally get off the hamster wheel of weight loss and into the driver's seat of your life.

I'VE GOT YOU, AND YOU'VE GOT THIS

I, for one, am proud of you for actually finishing this book. I mean, really, how often do we finish whole books these days? I know your journey is going to feel different from here on out, and I'm excited for you to put what you've learned into action. Remember to be gentle with yourself. Show yourself love and compassion throughout all the ebbs and flows that are going to come your way and enjoy life as much as possible while you try to crack the code on your new approach to health and wellness. Don't forget to celebrate yourself each step of the way—whether you're winning or failing and learning from your mistakes. Each day you prioritize your health and wellness will be another day you reinforce who you are, what is important to you, and what you are looking for in your life.

Each time you come to an inflection point, or you have to take a detour, or you have to make a decision, I want you to ask yourself: "Who would I be if no one was watching?

Let your transformation be about taking back control, claiming agency over your life, and having the courage to make the choices that feel right for you. Make the choice to live a life by design: to accept who you really are, to maximize it, and to share it with the world because after years of chaos with your body, you are now in the driver's seat and only you control the GPS.

So, are you ready to start . . . today?

Notes

1. Joachim Stoeber, "Perfectionism," in *Encyclopedia of Personality and Individual Differences*, ed. V. Zeigler-Hill and T. Shackelford (New York City: Springer Cham: 2016), doi. org/10.1007/978-3-319-28099-8_2027-1.
2. Rory Batchilder, "14 Signs Your Perfectionism Has Gotten out of Control," Westboro Counselling & Psychotherapy, February 21, 2018, rorybatchilder.com/1966-2.
3. *Cambridge Dictionary*, s.v. "calorie (*n*.)," dictionary.cambridge.org /dictionary/english/calorie.
4. *Cambridge Dictionary*, s.v. "metabolism (*n*.)," dictionary. cambridge.org/dictionary/english/metabolism.
5. Kris Gunnars, "10 Evidence-Based Health Benefits of Intermittent Fasting," Healthline, August 16, 2016, healthline.com/nutrition /10-health-benefits-of-intermittent-fasting.
6. Rudy Mawer, "Calorie Cycling 101: A Beginners Guide," Healthline, updated October 14, 2021, healthline.com/nutrition/calorie -cycling-101#TOC_TITLE_HDR_3.
7. Kris Gunnars, "Is Fructose Bad for You? The Surprising Truth," Healthline, April 23, 2018, healthline.com/nutrition/why-is -fructose-bad-for-you#section3.
8. Gunnars, "Is Fructose Bad for You?"
9. Helen West, "How to Speed Up Your Metabolism: 9 Easy Ways to Boost Your Metabolism Backed by Science," Healthline, July 27, 2018, healthline.com/nutrition/10-ways-to-boost-metabolism.

10. Harvard Health Publishing, "The Truth about Fats: The Good, the Bad, and the In-between," Harvard Health Publishing, August 13, 2018, health.harvard.edu/staying-healthy /the-truth-about-fats-bad-and-good.

11. Jessie Szalay, "Brown Rice: Health Benefits & Nutrition Facts," Livescience, October 3, 2018, livescience.com/50461-brown-rice -health-benefits-nutrition-facts.html.

12. Water Science School, "The Water in You: Water and the Human Body," USGS, usgs.gov/special-topic/water-science-school/science /water-you-water-and-human-body?qt-science_center_objects =0#qt-science_center_objects.

13. Kathleen M. Zelman, "6 Reasons to Drink Water," Nourish by WebMD, webmd.com/diet/features/6-reasons-to-drink-water#1.

14. Paige Waehner, "Everything You Need to Know about Cardio," Very Well Fit, August 2, 2019, verywellfit.com/everything-you -need-to-know-about-cardio-1229553.

15. "The Push/Pull/Legs Routine for Muscle Gains," Aston University, aston.ac.uk/sport/tips-information/the-push-pull-legs-routine -for-muscle-gains.

16. "Compound Exercises Have Many Benefits," Post Bulletin, November 6, 2012, postbulletin.com/sports/localsports/compound -exercises-have-many-benefits/article_3aef797b-88f0-5808-8b8e -8f2a1f98fa4b.html.

17. Paige Waehner, "Get Started with Weight Training," Very Well Fit, June 25, 2022, verywellfit.com/strength-4157137.

18. Mathias Wernbom, Jesper Augustsson, and Roland Thomeé, "The Influence of Frequency, Intensity, Volume and Mode of Strength Training on Whole Muscle Cross-Sectional Area in Humans," *Sports Medicine* 37, no. 3 (2007): 225-64, ncbi.nlm.nih.gov /pubmed/17326698.

19. Grant Tinsley, "7 Benefits of High-Intensity Interval Training (HIIT)," Healthline, June 2, 2017, healthline.com/nutrition/benefits-of-hiit.

20. Fara Rosenzweig, "What Is Tabata Training?" Active, February 1, 2018, active.com/fitness/articles/what-is-tabata-training.

21. Catherine Moore, "Positive Daily Affirmations: Is There Science behind It?" PositivePsychology, March 4, 2019, positivepsychology .com/daily-affirmations.

About the Author

SONIA JHAS is a TEDX speaker and an award-winning mindset and wellness expert. She is fired up by her mission to help people marry healthy living with a life lived well. Her special brand of inspiration and wisdom involves tried-and-true techniques that help people unlock lasting momentum and unapologetic self-fulfillment. Sonia's enthusiasm, sense of humor, and openness about her own journey have earned her a reputation as an unstoppable force in the wellness arena.

Happiness Starts... Today

HERE WE ARE, AT THE end of my book and the beginning of your journey. First of all, thank you—no, seriously, thank *you*—for making your way through *I'll Start Again Tomorrow: And Other Lies I've Told Myself*. I know how difficult it can be to show up for yourself and commit to the *real* work. And here you are, doing the thing! I'm so proud of you.

Let's stay in touch:

- @SoniaJhas
- Sonia Jhas
- @SoniaJhas
- @sonia_jhas

For speaking inquiries: booking@soniajhas.com

One final note:

 If *I'll Start Again Tomorrow: And Other Lies I've Told Myself* resonated with you, scan the QR code to the left and leave a review (if you want to!).

CPSIA information can be obtained
at www.ICGtesting.com
Printed in the USA
BVHW031236010223
657355BV00004B/12